Indian Head
Massage

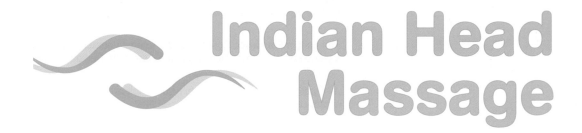

Indian Head Massage

Francesca Gould

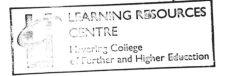
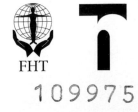

FHT

109975

Published in 2002 by:
Nelson Thornes Ltd
Delta Place
27 Bath Road
CHELTENHAM
GL53 7TH
United Kingdom

02 03 04 05 06 / 10 9 8 7 6 5 4 3 2 1

A catalogue record for this book is available from the British Library

ISBN 0 7487 6559 X

Illustrations by Oxford Designers and Illustrators and Angela Lumley
Page make-up by Florence Production Ltd

Printed and bound in Croatia by Zrinski

Contents

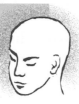

Preface

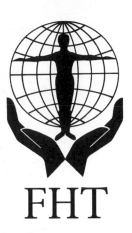

FHT

Indian head massage, although an ancient craft, is ideally suited to the needs of the twenty-first century. Stress-related illness is the major cause of the queues in our GPs' waiting rooms. Many in the established medical profession now acknowledge the benefits of complementary therapies such as Indian head massage in reducing stress, the underlying cause of a vast array of symptoms.

Indian head massage is one of the fastest growing of the new therapies. The level of relaxation that it is possible to achieve has to be seen, or experienced, to be believed. Many times we have witnessed clients, even in a busy exhibition hall, fall asleep after only the shortest of treatments. Its effectiveness lies in its simplicity and it is ideally suited to being offered as much in the workplace as the home, salon or clinic.

The Federation of Holistic Therapists, being the largest professional association for practitioners, welcomes this new publication. Learning a new holistic therapy is always both a daunting and exciting prospect and, as with all really effective treatments, looks easier to achieve than it really is. This essentially practical book will enable students to develop the skills necessary in a step-by-step fashion. The illustrations will help to refresh memories between formal teaching sessions and the questions will help to test for understanding. So whatever the background, whether as a complete beginner or practitioner experienced in other therapies, there is something of value to be found in these pages.

Jacqueline Palmer
Chief Executive, Federation of Holistic Therapists

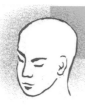

I have written this book for students undertaking professional Indian head massage courses such as the VTCT and ITEC qualifications.

Indian head massage is an extremely popular treatment. It can be carried out almost anywhere and the client does not need to remove any clothes! Not only holistic and beauty therapists working towards VTCT and ITEC qualifications but also people from hairdressing and nursing are showing great interest in learning this skill. I am sure it will not be long before the treatment is offered in many hairdressing shops, as well as beauty and holistic therapy centres.

The book is designed to be a workbook and there are tasks and questions throughout to test your knowledge. When completed they will make excellent revision notes for tests. At the back of the book you will find a fold-out section containing the Indian head massage routine, which will be a very useful 'quick glance' resource to help you practise the massage. I have also included a whole chapter on chakras and auras, as not only are they relevant to the Indian head massage treatments but they are in themselves subjects that my students and I have found fascinating. There are even some useful tips on how to see auras!

Francesca Gould
January 2002

Acknowledgements

I would like to thank my holistic therapy students 2000–2001, who gave me a great deal of support during the writing of this book.

I would also like to thank Amarjeet Bahamra from the Indian Head Massage Institute for his help and advice in the production of this book; it was most appreciated. Thanks to Caroline Gammon for being a great model and for her help with the massage routine.

The publishers would like to thank the following people for their help in producing this book:

Corel (NT) for Figure 4.8 on page 115 and Figure 4.10 on page 116; Martin Sookias for the photographs showing massage movements on pages 107–148; Heather Mole of VTCT and Helen Lewis of Warwickshire College for reviewing the manuscript and providing comments and recommendations, particularly on the design of the fold-out cover.

Cover image © Institute of Indian Head Massage, 38 Store Street, London WC1E 7DB www.indian headmassage.org. This book does not claim to be endorsed by the Institute.

Introduction to Indian Head Massage

1

HISTORY OF INDIAN HEAD MASSAGE

Indian head massage has been practised in India for over 5000 years.

It is based on the ancient Ayurvedic healing system in India. Ayurvedic medicine is a holistic healing system, which combines natural therapies and encompasses the mind, body and spirit. It strives to restore balance and inner harmony to the mind, body and spirit to improve the health of an individual.

> **Note**
>
> Ayurveda means 'the science of life'.

Indian women traditionally practise Indian head massage for the health benefits that the massage provides. Also, the hot climate is very drying to the hair, so women use oils during the massage to keep the hair shiny and in good condition. Different oils are used at various times of the year depending on the availability, cost and season. In south India there is an abundance of coconut trees so coconut oil is mostly used all year round. In the north there are a large quantity of mustard plants so mustard oil is mainly used all year round.

The skill is handed down from generation to generation and members of the family often give and receive head massages. Mothers will massage their babies every day and, between the ages of 3 and 6, children are massaged once or twice each week. Mothers will continue to give head massages to their children even when grown up. An expectant mother will be given a head massage up to the day the baby is born.

The massage not only has excellent physical effects but also helps with bonding and is a way of showing affection. After the age of 6, children are taught the skill of massage and will give and receive massage throughout life until old age.

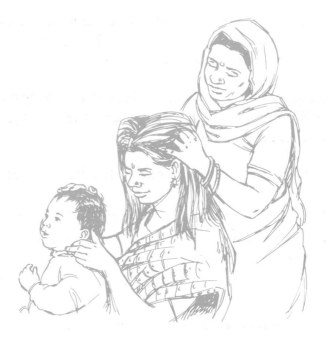

In India, before a couple are married they will receive massages. Various oils will be used that will make the skin and hair look healthy and help to relax the couple before the ceremony.

In holiday resorts around India there are head massage treatments on offer. If you visit a barber's shop in India, a head massage is always part of the service. In certain parts of India, barbers refer to head massage as *champi*.

Many men and women claim that it helps to prevent early greying and balding – although this has not yet been scientifically proven.

What is Indian head massage?

Indian head massage can help to relax, soothe or invigorate the receiver. It is a treatment that involves the therapist using their hands to knead, rub and squeeze the body's soft tissues, such as the muscles.

Oils such as coconut and almond can be used and may be applied to the face, neck and scalp. The oils help to keep the hair strong, healthy and lustrous.

Indian head massage treatment is becoming very popular in the West and has advantages over other massage treatments for the following reasons:

- Clients do not have to remove their clothes, unless they want to.
- It can be carried out almost anywhere.
- It can be carried out within a relatively short space of time compared to other holistic treatments.
- The massage can be performed with or without oils or creams.
- Little equipment is required, therefore it is an economical treatment to carry out.

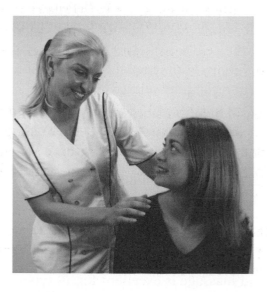

PHYSIOLOGICAL AND PSYCHOLOGICAL BENEFITS OF INDIAN HEAD MASSAGE

An Indian head massage treatment is very beneficial for physical and emotional health. It has the following benefits:

- It promotes total relaxation, as the massage helps to give a feeling of wellbeing and calm.
- The increased blood circulation to the head, neck and shoulders brings oxygen and nutrients, thus helping to improve the condition of the skin and to stimulate hair growth.
- The increased blood circulation to the brain means that more oxygen is delivered; this will help mental fatigue and improve concentration.
- The increased blood circulation will help to relieve stiffness in the neck and shoulders as oxygen and nutrients are brought to the area and waste products that have built up in the affected muscles are taken away.
- Massage relieves eyestrain and tension headaches as muscular tension is relieved.
- The increased lymphatic flow helps to get rid of toxins and other waste products, so aiding detoxification of the body.
- Massage helps with irritability and promotes sleep as the client feels more relaxed and calm.
- It breaks down fibrositic nodules, commonly known as 'knots', which develop from tension within the muscles.
- It triggers the release in the brain of chemicals called endorphins, which create a feeling of contentment and happiness.

STRESS

Indian head massage is excellent for all types of stress-related problems and an understanding of stress and its causes will help you to give your client a holistic treatment. For example, if your client is suffering from continual tension headaches, rather than just treating the headache, perhaps the client can be encouraged to take time to relax or to change their lifestyle in some way such as taking up exercise or adopting a healthier diet, or you may even be able to help them develop a more positive way of thinking that will alleviate stress and help to prevent the headaches.

Task 1.1

List the physical and emotional (psychological) benefits of Indian head massage.

Physical	Psychological
_____	_____
_____	_____
_____	_____
_____	_____
_____	_____
_____	_____
_____	_____
_____	_____

Note

It has been shown that people receiving any kind of healing treatment like Indian head massage have increased alpha waves in the brain. This is also a feature of people who are in a meditative state. This deep state of relaxation is associated with alleviated stress, improved breathing, lower blood cholesterol, better hormonal balance and increased immunity.

Cause of stress

Stress means different things to different people but generally it is a state we experience when there are demands placed on us and we do not feel that we have the ability to cope with them. Sometimes these demands can be stimulating and we cope well, as we feel able to deal with the demands and in control of the situation. Stress is generally thought of as a bad thing but it can often be positive – it may be needed to motivate and make us more effective and challenged.

Basically there are two types of stress. One is positive stress, such as that experienced by joggers, which they voluntarily place on themselves. Positive stress could be described as a high, excited tension, as when things are going your way in your job so you are achieving something. Negative stress, on the other hand, comes from, for example, sitting at a desk piled high with urgent papers and with many phones ringing all at once. Other causes of negative stress include bereavement, redundancy, moving house, pregnancy, financial difficulties and relationship breakup.

Personality traits largely decide which people are most vulnerable to the effects of stress. Competitive, ambitious over-achievers often tend to be stressed. These people can be impatient, hurried and highly conscious of time. People who are easy going and calm are less likely to become stressed. They may often appear patient and relaxed.

Many normally occurring stresses can be dealt with and we will recover from them without any serious ill effect. If stress levels are continually high, however, we become anxious and feel overloaded. Eventually, exhaustion and burnout occur. When stress becomes excessive it affects every system of the body as well as our minds. Stress is a contributory factor in almost every serious human illness. The more stressed you are the more likely you are to suffer from both physical and mental problems.

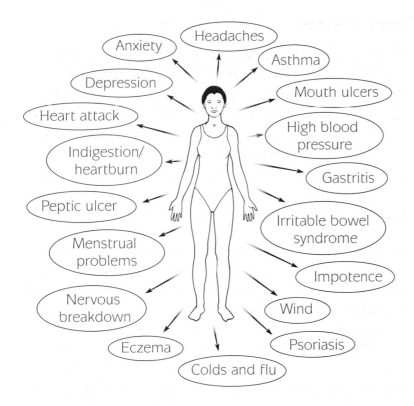

Men and women often respond differently to stress. Women become emotional and irritable, with headaches, irritable bowel syndrome, anxiety and depression (see diagram above). Men are more likely to suffer from high blood pressure.

The following advice can be given to someone suffering from negative stress.

- Become more assertive – learn to say no!
- Turn negative thoughts into positive ones. Negative thoughts never did anyone any good.
- Become more organised and set regular attainable goals. Tick them off as you achieve them.
- Write things down – it often helps to clear anxieties and fears from the mind.
- Take up a hobby or some sort of activity such as yoga or tai-chi – these are excellent for relaxation.
- Attend a stress management and relaxation course.

Stress sufferers may overeat, undereat, smoke or drink a lot of alcohol. They should be encouraged to reduce caffeine and alcohol intake and also to stop smoking. This will help to limit the amount of toxins being put into the body, which will help the body to deal more effectively with the effects of stress. A healthy diet is very important and sufferers should moderate their intake of refined sugar, found in cakes, biscuits and sweets. Regular exercise such as walking and swimming can also be of great help. Indian head massage treatments are an excellent way of reducing stress and will help to alleviate many of the symptoms.

HEALTHY BREATHING AND RELAXATION TECHNIQUES

For most people normal, everyday breathing tends to be shallow and rapid. It mostly involves the chest expanding out and then relaxing inwards. Deep breathing for relaxation is slow and deep, it involves using the diaphragm (see Chapter 2, page 91) and comes from the abdomen. Breathing, when done correctly, requires a person to inhale slowly through the nose and exhale out through the mouth; this prevents the throat from becoming dry. As air is inhaled the stomach should be allowed to move outwards. The diaphragm is pulled downwards, causing the lungs to draw in air to fill the space. The diaphragm will then relax, causing air to be expelled from the lungs and so we breathe out.

Slow, deep and rhythmic breathing triggers a relaxation response in the body. Some of these changes include a slower heart rate, muscular relaxation and a feeling of calmness. Relaxation exercises also trigger a relaxation response in the body.

Relaxation exercises

1. Either sit or lie down, and ensure you are comfortable. Clench both hands into fist shapes, hold for about 5 seconds and release.

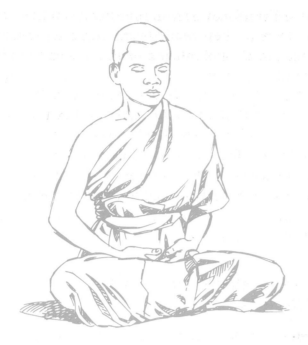

Now tense the muscles in the arms, hold for about 5 seconds and release. Work through the body, tightening the muscles over the front of the body, including the legs and face, then concentrating on the back of the body, until all muscles have been clenched and released.

This exercise should be repeated twice. It is good technique for releasing tension from muscles and so can help with headaches, aches and pains. It is excellent for relaxing the whole body.

2. Close your eyes and take several deep breaths. Begin releasing tension in the neck by rolling the head slowly from side to side. Allow tension to drain from the head, face and neck like melting wax. Feel the tension flowing out of the chest and arms. Continue this relaxation exercise working the upper body, then the stomach, lower back and buttocks. Most of the body should now be feeling heavy and relaxed.

Remove any tension from the legs, continuing to breath slowly. Imagine your legs are heavy and relaxed.

Note

Take in a deep breath as you carry out each hold and release exercise.

Note

The white, healing light is energy sent from the universe. In India it is called *prana*.

Visualise the flow of tension running down the calves. Now, concentrate on your feet and think about how they feel. Imagine the tension and pressure of walking flowing out of the feet.

Now imagine a white, warm, healing light penetrating the top of your head and flowing through the body, down your arms and legs and out through the hands and feet, taking away all tension and troubling thoughts. The warm light is freely flowing to heal and relax the body.

Visualisation

Visualisation is a powerful tool for helping to de-stress and relax both you and your client. Ensure you are comfortable and warm and then close your eyes.

Healing sanctuary

Imagine yourself walking along a country lane on a beautiful, warm day. You are feeling very happy and safe. You see a hot air balloon in a nearby field. As you reach the field you see a wooden gate. You open the gate and walk towards the balloon.

In this field you are only allowed to think of positive, happy thoughts, so you have to empty all of your problems and negative thoughts into the balloon's basket. When you have finished, the balloon with your problems floats away into the distance until it is no longer visible.

Now you look over to the other side of the field and see a wall of ivy. You walk up to it and use your hand to part the ivy, and then walk inside. This place is your private healing sanctuary. You can picture anything you like such as a room, cave, beach, etc. as long as you find it beautiful, calming and relaxing.

Stay there until you feel you have had enough healing and then walk back through the ivy, then through the field. Ensure you close the gate behind you and then walk back down the country lane....

This visualisation would be an excellent way to prepare and ground yourself prior to giving an Indian head massage.

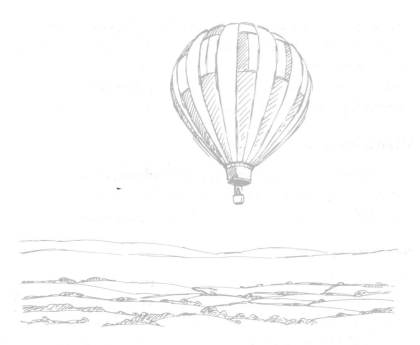

Ask yourself the following self-test questions:
1. How long has Indian head massage been practised in India?
2. What is the traditional reason why Indian women gave each other a head massage?
3. State ten benefits of receiving an Indian head massage.
4. What symptoms may a client show if they are suffering with stress?
5. How can an Indian head massage help to treat people suffering with symptoms of stress?
6. What is the correct way to breathe for relaxation?

Write down your answers on a sheet of paper. There are sample answers at the back of the book.

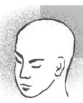

Anatomy and Physiology

Skin

The skin is a large organ and forms a protective, waterproof covering over the entire surface of the body. It is thinnest on the eyelids and thickest on the soles of the feet. The skin is continually shedding and renewing itself. It is made up of layers called the epidermis, dermis and subcutaneous layer.

EPIDERMIS

The upper portion of the skin consists of five layers and is known as the epidermis.

① Horny layer (stratum corneum)

The top layer of the epidermis is called the horny layer, and consists of flat, overlapping, **keratinised** cells. Keratin is a protein responsible for the hardening process (keratinisation) that cells undergo when they change from living cells with a nucleus to dead cells without a nucleus. Cells that have undergone keratinisation are therefore dead.

The keratinised cells help to prevent bacteria entering through the skin and protect the body from minor injury. Cells of the horny layer are continually being rubbed off the body by friction and are replaced by cells from the layers beneath. The shedding of dead skin cells is known as **desquamation**.

Note

About 80% of house dust consists of dead skin cells.

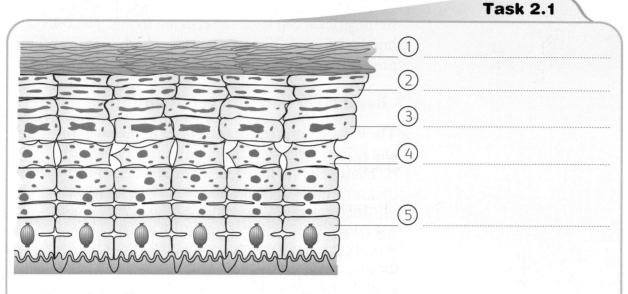

① ....
② ....
③ ....
④ ....
⑤ ....

Figure 2.1 *The epidermis*

Label the diagram in Figure 2.1, matching the numbers to the numbered terms on pages text on pages 12–14.

② Clear layer (stratum lucidum)

The clear layer is found below the horny layer and consists of dead, keratinised cells without a nucleus. The cells are transparent, which allows the passage of sunlight into the deeper layers. This layer is only found on the fingertips, the palms of the hands and the soles of the feet.

③ Granular layer (stratum granulosum)

The granular layer contains cells that have a granular appearance. As the cells die they fill with tiny granules called **keratohyalin** and so keratinisation begins to take place. This layer consists of living and dead cells.

④ **Prickle cell layer (stratum spinosum)**

In the prickle cell layer the cells are living. The cells interlock by arm-like fine threads, which give the cells a prickly appearance.

⑤ **Basal layer (stratum germinatum)**

The basal layer is the deepest layer in the epidermis and is in contact with the dermis directly beneath it. These cells are living, contain a nucleus and divide (mitosis) to make new skin cells. As new cells are produced they push older cells above them towards the surface of the skin, until they finally reach the horny layer. It takes 3–6 weeks for the skin cells to be pushed up from the basal layer to the horny layer.

Note

To help you remember the layers of the epidermis, depending on which names you need to learn, think of:

Happy – **h**orny	or	**Corny** – stratum **corn**eum
Clever – **cl**ear		**Lucy's** – stratum **luci**dum
Girls – **gr**anular		**Granny** – stratum **gran**ulosum
Pat – **p**rickle cell		**Spins** – stratum **spin**osum
Back – **b**asal		**Germs** – stratum **germ**inatum.

Skin pigmentation

Cells called **melanocytes** are found within the basal layer and produce granules of melanin. Melanin is responsible for the pigment (colour) of the skin and is stimulated by ultraviolet rays from the sun. This is why the skin develops a tan after sunbathing. Its function is to protect the deeper layers of the skin from damage.

Approximately 1 in every 10 basal cells is a melanocyte. Everyone has the same amount of melanocytes but produces varying quantities of melanin. This will determine the depth of skin colour. More melanin is produced in black skins than white skins, and this extra protection can help black skins to age more slowly than white skins.

DERMIS

Below the epidermis lies the dermis, which connects with the basal layer. It consists of two layers: the upper section is called the papillary layer and below it is the reticular layer.

The **papillary layer** contains small tubes called **capillaries**, which carry blood and lymph; there are also nerve endings. This layer provides nutrients for the living layers of the epidermis.

The **reticular layer** contains many connective tissue fibres. Collagen gives the skin strength and elastin gives the skin its elasticity. Wavy bands of tough collagen fibres restrict the extent to which the skin can be stretched, and elastic fibres return the skin back to shape after it has been stretched.

The dermis also contains nerves, hair follicles, sebaceous glands, sweat glands and erector pili muscles; these are known as **appendages**.

① **Erector pili muscles** are small muscles attached to the hair follicles. When we are cold the contraction of these muscles causes the hairs to stand on end. This results in the appearance of goose bumps. Air is trapped between the skin and hair and is warmed by the body heat. This helps to keep the body warm.

There are two types of sweat gland in the body: eccrine and apocrine glands.

Task 2.2

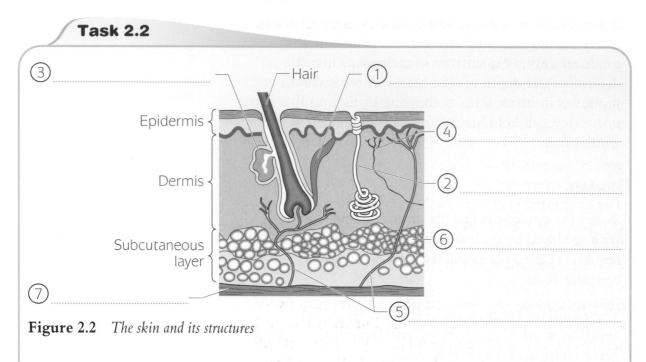

Figure 2.2   *The skin and its structures*

Label the diagram in Figure 2.2, matching the numbers to the numbered terms in the text on pages 15–17.

② **Eccrine glands** excrete sweat and are found all over the body. The sweat duct opens directly on to the surface of the skin through an opening called a pore. Sweat is a mixture of water, salt and toxins. Black skins contain larger and more numerous sweat glands than white skins.

Apocrine glands are found in the armpits, around the nipples and in the groin area. They secrete a milky substance. These glands are larger than eccrine glands and are attached to the hair follicle. Apocrine glands are controlled by hormones, becoming active at puberty. Body odour is caused by the breaking down of the apocrine sweat by bacteria. Substances called pheromones are present in this milky substance; the smell is thought to play a part in sexual attraction between individuals and the recognition of mothers by their babies.

Note

To help you remember the sweat glands think of **E** (eccrine glands) for **everywhere** and **A** (apocrine glands) for **armpits**.

③ **Sebaceous glands** are small, sac-like structures and produce a substance called sebum. Sebum is a fatty substance and is the skin's natural moisturiser. These glands are found all over the body but are more numerous on the scalp and areas of the face such as the nose, forehead and chin. Hormones control the activity of these glands and as we get older the secretion of sebum decreases, causing the skin to become drier. Sebum and sweat mix together on the skin to form an **acid mantle**. The **acid mantle** maintains the pH (acid/alkaline level) of the skin at 5.5–5.6; this helps to protect the skin from harmful bacteria. Some soaps can affect the acid mantle and cause irritation and drying of the skin.

Sensory and motor nerve endings – ④ **sensory nerve endings** are found all over the body but are particularly numerous on our fingertips and lips. These nerves will make us aware of feelings of pain, touch, heat and cold by sending messages through sensory nerves to the brain.

Messages are sent from the brain through **motor nerves**. Motor nerves will stimulate the sweat glands, erector pili muscles and sebaceous glands to carry out their functions.

⑤ **Blood vessels** – blood within these vessels provides the skin with oxygen and nutrients. The living cells of the skin produce waste products such as carbon dioxide and metabolic waste. These waste products pass from the cells and enter into the bloodstream to be taken away and removed by the body.

SUBCUTANEOUS LAYER

The subcutaneous layer is situated below the dermis. It consists of ⑥ **adipose tissue (fat)** and areolar tissue. The adipose tissue helps to protect the body against injury and acts as an insulating layer against heat loss, helping to keep the body warm. The areolar tissue contains elastic fibres, making this layer elastic and flexible. ⑦ **Muscle** is situated below the subcutaneous layer.

Task 2.3

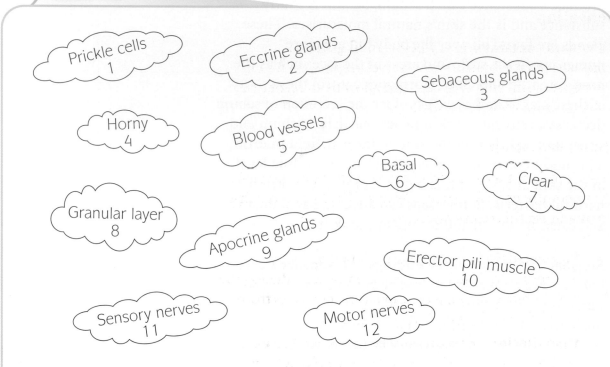

Prickle cells
1

Eccrine glands
2

Sebaceous glands
3

Horny
4

Blood vessels
5

Basal
6

Clear
7

Granular layer
8

Apocrine glands
9

Erector pili muscle
10

Sensory nerves
11

Motor nerves
12

Match the numbered phrases with the sentences below:

- Process of keratinisation takes place here ___
- Dead cells of this layer are rubbed off by friction ___
- Contracts causing hair to stand on end ___
- Layer found on palms of hands and soles of feet ___
- Send messages informing the brain about the sensations of pain, hot and cold ___
- Deepest layer in epidermis and in contact with the dermis ___
- Found all over the body and excrete sweat ___
- Stimulate sweat glands and sebaceous glands to carry out their functions ___
- Release a moisturising substance called sebum ___
- Living cells with a prickly appearance ___
- Release milky substance and found in armpits and groin area ___
- Bring supplies of oxygen and nutrients vital to skin ___

FUNCTIONS OF THE SKIN

Sensation

The skin contains sensory nerve endings that send messages to the brain. These nerves respond to touch, pressure, pain, cold and heat and allow us to recognise objects from their feel and shape.

Heat regulation

It is important for the body to have a constant internal temperature of 36.8 degrees Celsius (°C). The skin helps to maintain this temperature by:

- **Vasoconstriction** – this occurs when the body becomes cold. The blood vessels constrict reducing the flow of blood through the capillaries. Heat loss from the surface of the skin is therefore reduced.

- **Vasodilation** – this occurs when the body becomes too hot. The capillaries expand and the blood flow increases; this allows heat to be lost from the body by radiation.

- **Goose bumps** – contraction of the erector pili muscle when we are cold causes the hairs to stand on end, keeping a layer of warm air close to the body. This was probably of more use to our ancestors, who were generally hairier.

- **Shivering** – shivering when we are cold helps to warm the body, as the contraction of the muscles produces heat within the body.

- **Sweating** – in hot conditions the rate of sweat production increases. The eccrine glands excrete sweat on to the skin surface and so heat is lost as the water evaporates from the skin.

Absorption

The skin is largely waterproof and absorbs very little, although certain substances are able to pass through the

Note

A good way of remembering the functions of the skin is the words SHAPES VD.

S – **s**ensation

H – **h**eat regulation

A – **a**bsorption

P – **p**rotection

E – **e**xcretion

S – **s**ecretion

VD – **v**itamin **D** formation.

basal layer. Essential oils can pass through the hair follicles and into the bloodstream. Certain medications such as hormone replacement therapy can be given through patches placed on the skin. Ultraviolet rays from the sun are also able to penetrate through the basal layer.

Protection

The skin protects the body by keeping harmful bacteria out and provides a covering for all the organs inside. It also protects underlying structures from the harmful effects of ultraviolet (UV) light. The other functions of the skin also help to protect the body.

Excretion

Eccrine glands excrete sweat on to the skin's surface. Sweat consists of 99.4% water, 0.4% toxins and 0.2% salts.

Secretion

Sebum is a fatty substance secreted from the sebaceous gland on to the skin's surface. It keeps the skin supple and helps to waterproof it.

Vitamin D

The UV rays from the sun penetrate through the skin's layers and activate a chemical found in the skin called ergosterol, which changes into vitamin D. Vitamin D is essential for healthy bones and deficiency can cause rickets, a condition in which the bones are malformed.

EFFECTS OF MASSAGE ON THE SKIN

- The circulation is improved and so fresh blood brings nutrients to the sebaceous glands; therefore sebum production is increased. More sebum helps to make the skin soft and supple.

- The sweat glands become more active and so more sweat is excreted. Toxins such as urea and other waste products are eliminated from the body in this way.

Note

The palms of the hands and soles of the feet do not have sebaceous glands.

Fill in the gaps in the following text.

- _____ nerve endings respond to touch, pressure and pain. They send the information to the brain.
- It is important for the body temperature to remain at _____.
- To reduce heat loss from the skin the blood vessels _____. This is known as vasoconstriction.
- When the body becomes too hot the capillaries dilate so heat can be lost. This is known as _____.
- Goose bumps are caused by the contraction of the _____ _____ muscles.
- Shivering helps to _____ the body because of the contraction of the muscles.
- Sweating helps to _____ the body as heat is lost as the sweat evaporates.
- The skin can absorb certain substances, including the following: _____ _____, _____ and _____ _____.
- Sweat consists of water, _____ and _____
- A fatty substance called _____ is secreted on to the skin's surface.
- Vitamin ___ production is stimulated by the penetration of UV rays through the skin.

- Massage also causes the top layer of dead skin cells to be shed (desquamation), which improves the condition of the skin, giving it a healthy glow.

- The sensory nerve endings can either be soothed or stimulated, depending on the massage movements used.

- When massage and essential oils are used together the skin's health and appearance can be greatly improved.

SKIN AGEING

When a person is in their early twenties the skin should be at its best. In the late twenties and early thirties fine lines appear on the skin's surface, especially around the eyes where the skin is thinner.

After 40 years hormone activity in the body slows down so the sebaceous glands produce less sebum and the skin becomes increasingly drier. Lines and wrinkles appear on the surface. Wrinkling is due to changes in the collagen and elastin fibres of the connective tissue. The collagen fibres in the dermis begin to decrease in number, stiffen and break apart. The elastin fibres lose some of their elasticity and break down, so that when the skin is stretched it does not immediately return to its original state when stretching stops. In people who are regularly exposed to ultraviolet light or who smoke, the loss of elasticity of the skin is greatly accelerated. Constant facial expressions cause **crow's feet** to be found at the sides of the eyes.

In the late fifties brown patches of discoloured skin called lentigines (liver spots) may appear because of an increase in the size of some melanocytes. Liver spots are commonly seen around the temple areas of the face and on the backs of the hands. The blood flow to the skin is reduced and the rate of mitosis in the basal layer slows down. The horny layer is therefore thinner, making the skin more fragile. Dilated capillaries appear, especially on the cheeks and nose.

Sebaceous glands decrease in size, which leads to dry and cracked skin. The sweat glands are less active and loss of subcutaneous fat often occurs. The hair growth slows down and a decrease in the number of functioning melanocytes results in grey hairs. The skin of elderly people heals poorly and becomes more susceptible to infection and also skin cancer.

List five changes that take place in the skin as it ages.

1. _____

2. _____

   _____

3. _____

4. _____

5. _____

   _____

Factors affecting the condition of the skin

Ageing of the skin may occur naturally or it may prematurely age because of various factors, including heredity, environment (perhaps work outside in all weathers), inadequate diet, smoking or ill health (see Figure 2.3, page 27).

Diet

The best nutritional recommendation to ensure healthy skin is to eat a well balanced diet. The Western diet generally contains the essential vitamins and minerals required for a healthy skin. These include vitamins A, B_3 (niacin) and C. Vitamin A helps to control the rate of keratinisation in the skin and so deficiency of this vitamin can result in dry skin. If the diet is deficient in vitamin B_3 a disease called pellagra can occur; one of its features is dermatitis. Vitamin C is required by the body to produce collagen and deficiency of this vitamin can also lead to dermatitis.

Alcohol is not harmful to the skin in moderation but large amounts dilate the blood vessels and over time may weaken the capillary walls and lead to broken capillaries and redness; this can often be seen on the face. Alcohol also dehydrates the skin by drawing water from the tissues and robbing the body of vitamins B and C, which are required for a healthy skin.

Caffeine is found in tea, coffee and some soft fizzy drinks. In moderate doses it will cause no harm but excessive amounts can interfere with the absorption of vitamins and minerals, which can result in an unhealthy skin.

Sunlight

Ultraviolet radiation from the sun penetrates into the dermis of the skin and causes damage. It causes dehydration and also interferes with the structure of the collagen and elastin fibres. The skin loses its strength and elasticity, resulting in severe wrinkling and sagging, especially noticeable in people who spend a great deal of time in the sun.

Smoking

Smoking interferes with cell respiration and slows down the blood circulation, as nicotine is a vasoconstrictor. This makes it harder for nutrients to reach the skin cells and for waste products to be eliminated. Cigarette smoking also releases a chemical that destroys vitamin C. This interferes with the production of collagen and so contributes to premature ageing. People who have smoked for a long time will generally look 10 years older than non-smokers of the same age.

Medication

Certain medications taken by mouth can lead to skin dehydration, fluid retention or swelling of the tissues – steroids are an example. Hydrocortisone creams are applied externally and are used to treat skin conditions such as psoriasis and dermatitis. The cream should be used for short lengths of time and in small quantities otherwise thinning of the skin may result.

Note

Over 80% of wrinkling of the skin is due to sunlight exposure.

Antibiotics can cause temporary drying of the skin, although it will improve after the course of drugs has finished.

Taking the contraceptive pill can cause a condition known as chloasma. Areas of increased pigmentation occur on the skin, usually on the face.

Environmental

The moisture content of the epidermis can be affected by factors such as central heating, which creates a dry environment. This causes moisture to be lost from the epidermis and can lead to dehydration.

Air pollution from industry, car fumes, etc. harms the skin and causes dehydration.

If a person alternates between a cold and a warm environment the capillaries contract and dilate to adapt to that particular temperature. The capillary walls become weak and this leads to permanently **dilated capillaries**, also called **thread veins**. These can commonly be seen on the cheeks and nose. There are also many other causes of dilated capillaries.

SKIN TYPES

Skin types vary from person to person and can be described as being normal, dry, oily, combination, sensitive, dehydrated or mature. Essential oils can be chosen to suit each individual skin type.

Normal

This skin type will look healthy, clear and fresh. It is often seen in children, as external factors and ageing have not yet affected the condition of the skin, although the increased activity of hormones at puberty may cause the skin to become greasy. A normal skin type will look neither oily or dry and will have a fine, even texture. The pores are small and the skin's elasticity is good so it feels soft and firm to the touch. It is usually free of spots and blemishes.

Dry

This skin type is thin and fine and dilated capillaries can often be seen around the cheek and nose areas. The skin will feel and look dry because little sebum is being produced and it is also lacking in moisture. This skin type will often tighten after washing and there may be some dry, flaky patches. There will be no spots or comedones (blackheads) and no visible open pores. This skin type is prone to premature wrinkling, especially around the eyes, mouth and neck.

Task 2.6

Fill in the gaps in the following text.

- Vitamin ____ is required by the body to produce collagen.
- Excessive alcohol intake can lead to weakening of the _____ walls.
- UV rays cause _____ of the skin and also damage the structure of the _____ and _____ fibres.
- Smoking causes a chemical to be released that destroys vitamin____ .
- Long-term smokers are more prone to _____ ageing than non-smokers.
- Long-term use of hydrocortisone creams can cause _____ of the skin.
- While using antibiotics the skin can become _____.
- Central heating and air pollution can lead to the skin becoming _____.
- If the skin alternates between cold and warm environments, damage to the capillaries may result which leads to permanently dilated capillaries called _____ _____.

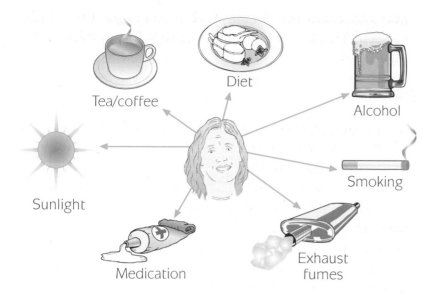

Figure 2.3 *Factors affecting the skin*

Oily

This skin type will look shiny, dull and slightly yellowish (sallow) in colour because of the excess sebum production. Oily skin is coarse, thick and will feel greasy. Enlarged pores can be seen; these are due to the excess production and build-up of sebum. Open pores can let in bacteria, which cause spots and infections. Blocked pores often lead to comedones (blackheads). Oily skin tends to age more slowly, as the grease absorbs some of the UV rays and so can protect against its damaging effects. The sebum also helps to keep the skin moisturised and prevents drying.

Combination

With this skin type there will be areas of dry, normal and greasy skin. Usually the forehead, nose and chin are greasy and are known as the T zone. The areas around the eyes and cheeks are usually dry and may be sensitive.

Sensitive

This skin type is often dry, transparent and reddens easily when touched. Dilated capillaries may be present, especially on the cheeks, which gives the face a high, red colour known as couperose skin. Hereditary factors may be a cause of sensitive skin. A skin that is sensitive may be easily irritated by certain substances so care should be taken when choosing products for this type. If a white skin is sensitive to a product it will show as a reddened area but on black skin it will show up as a darkened area.

Dehydrated

This skin type lacks moisture and so is dehydrated. The causes include illness, medication, too much sun, dieting and working in a dry environment with low humidity, such as an air-conditioned office. Sebum helps to prevent evaporation of water from the skin, so when insufficient sebum is produced, moisture is lost from the skin. The skin feels and looks dry and tight. There may be flaking and fine lines present on the skin. Dilated capillaries are also common with this skin type.

Mature

This skin type is dry as the sebaceous and sweat glands become less active. The skin may be thin and wrinkles will be present. There are usually dilated capillaries, often around the nose and cheek areas. The bone structure can become more prominent as the adipose and supportive tissue become thinner. Muscle tone is often poor so the contours of the face become slack. Because of the poor blood circulation, waste products are removed less quickly so the skin may become puffy and pale in colour. Liver spots may also appear on the face and hands. The cause of this skin type is ageing and altered hormone activity.

SKIN DISEASES AND DISORDERS

Skin diseases and disorders can be classified as bacterial infections, viral infections, fungal infections, infestations, allergies and non-infectious conditions. Some infections, such as ringworm and athlete's foot, can be caught by direct contact with an infected person. Infections can also be caught by indirect contact with contaminated items such as towels, coins, door handles, crockery, etc., which can store germs such as bacteria.

Write the characteristics of each skin type into the table below.

Skin type	Brief description
Normal	
Dry	
Oily	
Combination	
Sensitive	
Dehydrated	
Mature	

Bacterial infections

Bacteria are single-celled organisms and can multiply very quickly. They are capable of breeding outside the body so can be caught easily by direct contact or by touching a contaminated article.

There are two types of bacteria, pathogenic (harmful) and non-pathogenic (harmless). Infections occur when harmful bacteria enter the skin through broken skin or hair follicles. The most common are listed below. However, you should be aware that 'itis' simply means inflammation and that not all types of, for example, conjunctivitis are infectious. Allergic conjunctivitis is just a form of hay fever.

Boils

A boil is an infection of the hair follicle, which begins as a tender, red lump and develops into a painful pustule containing pus. It extends deep into the skin's tissue. Once a head is formed the pus is discharged, leaving a space, and so scarring of the skin often remains after the boil has healed. Poor general health and inadequate diet are factors increasing the chances of developing a boil. Sufferers are treated with antibiotics. Boils are infectious so the area affected should be avoided during massage treatment. Clients should be referred to their doctor if a boil appears on the upper lip or in the nose and boils can be dangerous if they occur near to the eyes or the brain. Carbuncles are a group of boils involving several hair follicles.

Styes

A stye is a small boil on the edge of the eyelid and is caused by an infection of the follicle of an eyelash. The area becomes inflamed, swollen and there may be pus present. Styes are infectious and generally occur when a person is in poor health or has an inadequate diet.

Conjunctivitis

This is inflammation of the conjunctiva, the membrane covering the eye. The inner eyelid and eyeball appear red and sore. It is caused by a bacterial infection following irritation to the eye, such as grit or dust that enter the eye, and is further aggravated by rubbing. Pus is often present and may ooze from the area. Conjunctivitis is infectious and cross-infection can occur through using contaminated towels or tissues.

Impetigo

This infection begins when bacteria invade a cut, cold sore or other broken skin. It can be seen as weeping blisters that form golden/yellow coloured crusts. The area around the crusts is inflamed and red. Impetigo is highly infectious and spreads quickly on the surface of the skin. Usually the outbreaks are among children and often go hand in hand with lice infestations. If this condition is suspected the sufferer must be referred to the doctor and treated with antibiotics.

Folliculitis

This is a bacterial infection of the hair follicles and sebaceous glands. The area infected is usually red and inflamed. It is infectious, so should be avoided during massage treatment.

Viral infection

Although very small, viruses are responsible for a great deal of human disease. They are protein-coated particles of RNA or DNA. Cells in the body are taken over by invading viruses and so break down. Viruses need living cells in which to live and multiply – they cannot live outside their host. Many viruses take up residence along nerve pathways, which accounts for the pain associated with many viral infections such as shingles. They can be transmitted by direct and indirect contact.

Cold sores

Cold sores are a common skin infection caused by the herpes simplex virus. It is usually passed on in early childhood, probably after being kissed by someone with a cold sore. The virus passes through the skin, travels up a nerve and lies dormant at a nerve junction. When the virus is stimulated it will travel back down the nerve and

Fungal infections

Fungi are microscopic plants and the spores reproduce by the process of cell division. Fungal infections often affect keratinised, dead tissue such as the nails and skin.

Ringworm (tinea corporis)

Ringworm is a fungal infection, not caused by a worm, and is sometimes caught through touching animals. It affects the horny layer of the skin and shows itself as red, scaly, circular patches which spread outwards. The centre of the patch heals, forming a ring shape. It usually appears on the trunk of the body, the limbs and the face. Ringworm is highly infectious so the area must be avoided during massage treatment and the client should be referred to their GP.

Scalp ringworm (tinea capitis)

Scalp ringworm infects the epidermis and forms grey, scaly areas. There is also breakage of hairs. It is infectious and massage over the affected area must be avoided.

Ringworm of the beard (tinea barbae)

There may be scaly patches, with partial hair loss in the affected areas. Although uncommon, it is infectious, so should be avoided during massage treatment.

Infestations

Animal parasites also cause disorders of the human skin.

Scabies

The scabies mite burrows into and lays its eggs in the horny layer of the skin. It can affect most areas of the body, although it is commonly found in the webs between the fingers and in the crease of the elbow. There is a 4–6 week incubation period before the outbreak. The female mite leaves a trail of eggs and excrement in the skin, which appears as wavy greyish lines. The condition

> **Note**
>
> Athlete's foot (*tinea pedis*) is a fungal infection affecting the feet.

Fill in the table below.

	Brief description	Is it infectious?
Ringworm (*Tinea corporis*)		
Scalp ringworm (*Tinea capitis*)		
Ringworm of the beard (*Tinea barbae*)		

is very itchy and highly infectious. No massage treatment should be given and the client should consult their doctor.

Hair lice

This parasite lives in hair, preferably clean, and feeds off the host's blood. The female lays 300 eggs each day and attaches them to hair close to the scalp. This condition is itchy and so infection can occur through scratching. No massage treatment should be given, as the condition is highly infectious.

Pigmentation disorders

Chloasma

This condition shows itself as patches of increased pigmentation on areas of the skin, often the face. The cause can be due to sunburn, pregnancy and the contraceptive pill. Chloasma is not infectious and massage treatment can be carried out.

Fill in the table below.

	Brief description	Is it infectious?
Scabies		
Hair lice		

Vitiligo

This condition shows itself as a complete loss of colour in areas of the skin. The affected areas have either lost their pigment or were never pigmented. The lightened patches of skin are very sensitive to sunlight and burn easily. The cause of vitiligo is unknown. It is not infectious and massage treatment can be carried out.

Albinism

In this condition, the skin is unable to produce the pigment melanin. The skin, hair and eyes all lack colour. Albinism is not infectious and massage treatment can be given.

Freckles (ephelides)

Freckles show themselves as small, pigmented areas of skin. The UV rays from sunlight stimulate the production of melanin and therefore either darken freckles or create new ones. Freckles are not infectious and can be worked over during massage.

Lentigo (plural – lentigines)

These are also known as liver spots. Although larger than freckles, they are also simply pigmented areas of skin, but lentigines do not darken when exposed to UV rays. They are usually slightly raised and brown in colour and are commonly seen on the face and hands. They are not infectious and can be worked over during massage.

Naevus (plural – naevi)

A naevus is a birthmark, often found on the face or neck. It can vary in size and is usually purplish pink in colour. It is not infectious and massage can be given over the affected area.

Port wine stain

This is caused by large areas of dilated capillaries, usually reddish in colour. Most occur on the head or sometimes the neck and face. They are not infectious and massage can be given over the affected area.

Skin allergies

Allergies

An allergy is an abnormal response by the body's immune system to a foreign substance (allergen). Some people can react to ordinary substances, normally harmless to most people. Irritation to the skin causes some of its cells release histamine, causing the skin to become warm, red and swollen.

It is advisable to give an allergy test to someone with sensitive skin; otherwise there may be a reaction to the essential oils or carrier oils. You should also ensure that

Task 2.12

Fill in the table below.

	Brief description	Is it infectious?
Chloasma		
Vitiligo		
Albinism		
Freckles (ephelides)		
Lentigo		
Naevus		
Port wine stain		

the client is not allergic to wheat or nuts if you intend to use wheatgerm or carrier oils extracted from nuts. An irritated skin due to an allergy is not infectious, but it is advisable not to massage over the affected area.

Hives (urticaria)

Urticaria is an allergic skin condition often called nettle rash or hives. A red rash develops that is very itchy and disappears completely within minutes or gradually over a number of hours. There are numerous causes of urticaria; it can occur as an allergic response to substances such as certain foods and drugs. It can also be caused by heat, cold, sunlight, scabies, insect bites and contact with plants. This condition is not infectious but it is advisable not to work over the affected area during massage treatment.

Dermatitis

Dermatitis is an inflammation of the skin caused by contact with external substances. Common irritants are detergents and dyes but materials such as nylon, wool and chemicals found in perfumes can produce allergic reactions that can lead to dermatitis. Certain metals such as nickel found in watchstraps, earrings and bra hooks can irritate the skin and lead to dermatitis in sensitive people. Symptoms include erythema, itching and flaking of the skin and in severe cases blisters can develop. Although the condition isn't infectious it is advisable not to work over the affected area until it has cleared up.

Eczema

Eczema used to be considered to be different from dermatitis but it now generally accepted that both terms may be used to describe the same condition. Eczema is inflammation of the skin and features itchy, dry, scaly red patches. Small blisters may burst, causing the skin to weep. Hereditary factors or external irritants such as detergents, cosmetics and soaps can cause eczema. Internal irritants such as dairy products can also be a trigger. This condition is not infectious, although it is advisable to avoid working over the affected areas during massage treatment, especially if there is weeping or bleeding.

Task 2.13

Fill in the table below.

	Brief description	Is it infectious?
Allergies		
Hives (urticaria)		
Dermatitis		
Eczema		

Sebaceous gland disorders

Whiteheads (milia)

If skin keratinises over the hair follicle it causes sebum to accumulate and become trapped in the hair follicle. A whitehead can be seen as a small white spot, which often accompanies dry skin. This condition is not infectious and can be massaged over.

Blackheads (comedones)

Blackheads occur when sebum becomes trapped in a hair follicle. Keratinised (dead) cells mix with the sebum and form a plug. The head of the comedo becomes black in colour because it combines with the oxygen in the air (oxidises). Comedones generally occur on greasy skin types and are not infectious. The affected area can be massaged over.

Acne vulgaris

Acne is a common complaint and usually affects teenagers. It is caused by an overproduction of sebum, usually due to stimulation of the sebaceous glands by hormones called testosterone and progesterone. During adolescence the levels of these sex hormones rise. The sebum, along with dead skin cells, becomes trapped in the openings of the sebaceous glands and, if they become infected, red and swollen spots will appear. Blackheads (comedones) also form and, if they become infected, the typical red and swollen spot appears. The spots are mainly found on the face, neck and back. Acne is not infectious but it is advisable for the client to consult their doctor before massage treatment if the acne is severe.

Rosacea

This condition is often referred to as acne rosacea. It mainly affects people over the age of 30 and is more common in women than men. Rosacea affects the nose, cheeks and forehead, giving a flushed, reddened appearance. The blood vessels, which are dilated in these areas, produce a butterfly shape. Pus-filled spots may appear and the affected area may also become lumpy, because of swollen sebaceous glands. Causes include eating spicy or hot food, drinking alcohol and stress. It is not an infectious condition but care needs to be taken when massaging over the affected areas. It is wise to avoid the area if a client has a severe case of rosacea.

Seborrhoea

This is a condition where the sebaceous glands release excessive amounts of sebum. It usually occurs during puberty because of the hormonal changes taking place in the body. There are open pores and the skin appears thick and greasy. Blackheads (comedones) and spots may also occur. It is not infectious and gentle massage treatment can be given.

Skin disorders involving abnormal growth

Psoriasis

In people with psoriasis the skin cells reproduce too quickly in certain areas of the skin. This results in thickened patches of skin, which are red, dry, itchy and covered in silvery scales. Psoriasis may be mild and only affect the elbows and knees or may cover the whole body, including the scalp. The cause is unknown although the condition tends to be hereditary and stress can be a factor. Psoriasis is not infectious so massage treatment can be given providing there is no bleeding or weeping and the client will not feel any discomfort.

Skin tags

Skin tags can affect most parts of the body, often the neck. They are made of loose fibrous tissue, which protrudes out from the skin, and are mainly brown in colour. They are harmless and are not infectious.

Fill in the table below.

	Brief description	Is it infectious?
Whiteheads (milia)		
Blackheads (comedones)		
Acne vulgaris		
Acne rosacea		
Seborrhoea		

Removal of skin tags can be carried out by a doctor or certain beauty clinics. It is advisable not to work over the skin tags as it may be uncomfortable for the client.

Skin cancer

There are three main types of skin cancer, named for the types of skin cell from which they develop.

Basal cell carcinoma and squamous cell carcinoma

Basal cell and squamous cell carcinomas account for 95% of all skin cancers. They are usually found on areas of the body often exposed to the sun, such as the face, neck, arms and hands. These cancers are often painless and begin as small, shiny, rounded lumps, which form into ulcers as they enlarge. They appear to be brought on by UV light and are usually seen in fair-skinned people. They are not infectious but should be avoided during massage treatment.

Melanoma

A melanoma is a skin growth due to overactivity of the melanocytes, usually caused by excessive exposure to the sun. Melanocyte overactivity may be benign, as in a mole, or malignant as in a malignant melanoma. Although rare and not infectious, malignant melanomas are extremely dangerous. They can occur anywhere on the body but often at the site of a mole. They are usually irregular in outline, patchy in colour, itchy or sore and may bleed. They spread very quickly and need prompt medical attention.

The danger signs to look out for are:

- the appearance of a new mole
- a mole that gets bigger
- a mole that bleeds, itches or ulcerates
- a mole that gets darker or lighter in colour.

Fill in the table below.

	Brief description	**Is it infectious?**
Psoriasis		
Skin tags		
Basal and squamous cell carcinomas		
Melanoma		

Hair

Most of the body is covered by hairs, with the exception of the palms of the hands and the soles of the feet. Hairs mainly consist of the protein keratin and grow out from follicles. Follicles are deep pits that extend into the dermis. Hairs help to keep the body warm and are also a form of protection. The eyelashes prevent substances from entering the eyes and the hairs that line the nose and ears help to trap dust and bacteria.

Note

A straight follicle will produce a straight hair, a curly follicle a curly hair.

Task 2.16

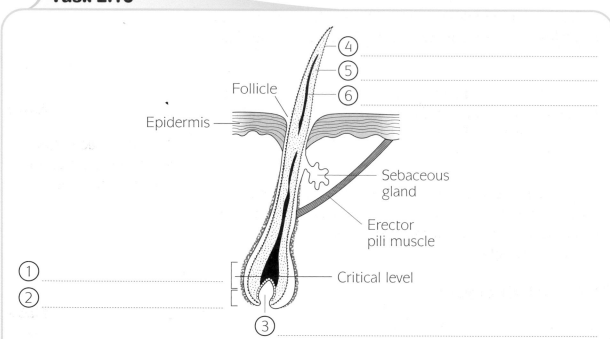

Follicle

Epidermis

Sebaceous gland

Erector pili muscle

Critical level

Figure 2.4 *A hair and its follicle*

Label the diagram in Figure 2.4, matching the numbers to the numbered terms in the text on pages 46–47.

The **bulb** ① is found at the base of the hair and has an upper and lower part. The **matrix** ② is the lower part of the bulb and this is where cell division takes place to create the hair. When cells reach the upper part of the bulb they quickly fill with keratin and die.

Melanin can be found in the upper part of the bulb and will determine the colour of hair. The hair bulb surrounds the **dermal papilla** ③, an area containing many blood vessels, which provides the necessary nutrients needed for hair growth.

The hair is made up of three layers known as the cuticle, cortex and medulla.

The **cuticle** ④ is the outer part of the hair and consists of a single layer of scale-like cells. These cells overlap rather like tiles on a roof. No pigment is contained within this layer.

The **cortex** ⑤ lies inside the cuticle and forms the bulk of the hair. It contains melanin, which determines the colour of the hair. The cortex helps to give strength to the hair.

The **medulla** ⑥ is the inner part of the hair and is not always present. Air spaces in the medulla determine the colour tone and sheen of the hair because of the reflection of light.

Types of hair growth

There are different types of hair growth:

- **Lanugo hair** is the hair found on the fetus and is usually shed by about the eighth month of pregnancy.
- **Vellus hair** is soft and downy and is found all over the body except on the palms and soles of the feet.
- **Terminal hair** is longer, coarser and the follicles are deeper than vellus hair. These hairs can be found on the head, eyebrows and eyelashes, under the arms and in the pubic region.

> **Note**
>
> The number and distribution of hair follicles are the same in both sexes.

> **Note**
>
> Hereditary factors will determine the specific hair growth patterns.

> **Note**
>
> Hormones are responsible for stimulating the growth of the hairs so will determine the quantity, thickness and distribution of hair on the body.

LIGAMENTS

Ligaments consist of bands of strong, fibrous connective tissue, silvery in appearance .They prevent dislocation by holding the bones across joints, but stretch slightly to allow movement.

TENDONS

Tendons consist of white, strong, almost inelastic, fibrous bands. Most muscles are attached to bones by tendons. They vary in length and thickness. When a muscle contracts, the force transmitted through the tendon creates movement at the bone. An example of a tendon is the Achilles tendon that attaches the calf muscle to the heel.

THE BONES OF THE SKELETON

Bones of the skull and face

① **Frontal bone** – one frontal bone forms the forehead.

② **Parietal bone** – two parietal bones form the sides and top of the skull.

③ **Temporal bone** – two temporal bones are found at the sides of the skull under the parietals.

④ **Occipital bone** – one occipital bone forms the back of the skull.

⑤ **Zygomatic bone** – two zygomatic bones form the cheekbones.

⑥ **Maxilla** – the maxilla forms the upper part of the jaw.

⑦ **Mandible** – the mandible forms the lower part of the jaw. It is the only movable bone of the skull.

⑧ **Ethmoid bone** – one ethmoid bone helps to form the eye socket and nasal cavities.

⑨ **Sphenoid bone** – one sphenoid bone helps to form the base of the skull.

⑩ **Nasal bone** – two nasal bones form the bridge of the nose.

> **Note**
>
> Remember:
>
> **Ligaments** attach bone to bone
>
> **Tendons** attach muscle to bone.

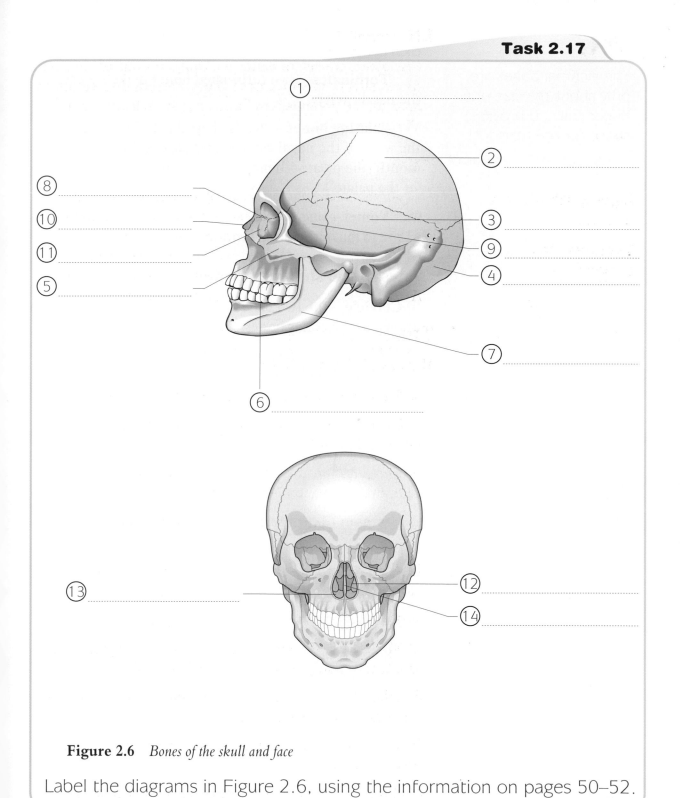

Figure 2.6 *Bones of the skull and face*

Label the diagrams in Figure 2.6, using the information on pages 50–52.

⑪ **Lacrimal bone** – two lacrimal bones make up part of each eye socket.

Note

The lacrimal bones are only about the size of a finger nail and provide space for the tear duct.

⑫ **Turbinates** – two turbinated bones make up part of the nasal cavity.

⑬ **Palatine bones** – two L-shaped palatine bones form the walls of the naval cavities and part of the roof of the mouth (the palate – hence the name 'palatine', meaning 'of the palate').

⑭ **Vomer** – one vomer extends upwards from the hard palate to make the nasal septum.

Bones of the shoulder girdle

① **Clavicle** – the two clavicles are long slender bones also known as the collar bones.

② **Scapula** – the two scapulae are large, triangular, flat bones also known as the shoulder blades.

Task 2.18

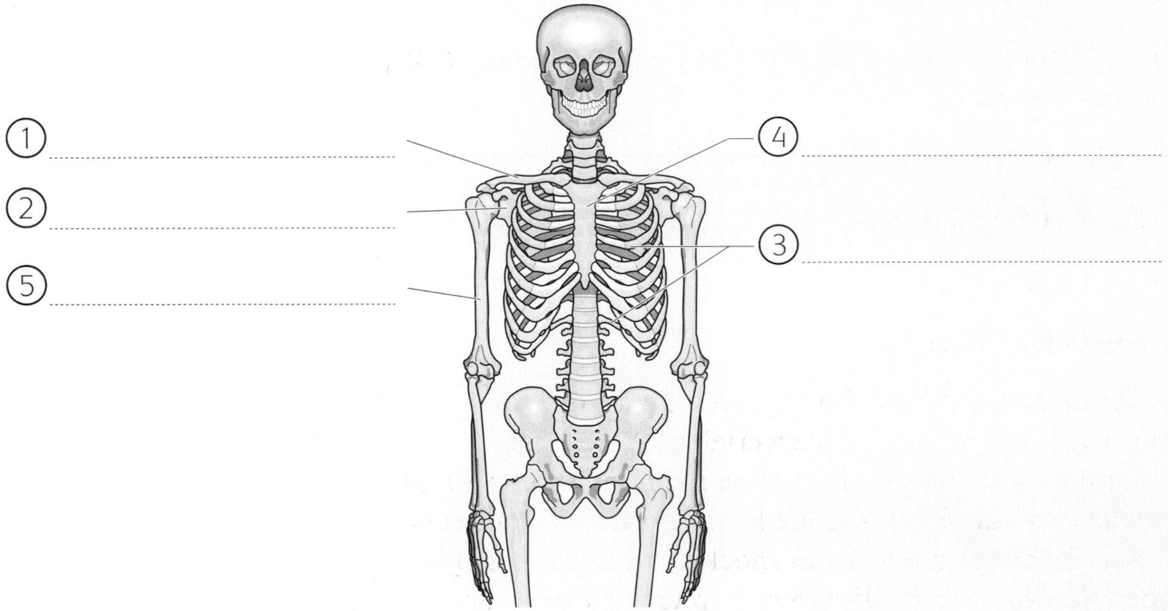

1 ....

2 ....

5 ....

4 ....

3 ....

Figure 2.7 *Bones of the upper body*

Label the diagrams in Figure 2.7, using the information on pages 52–53.

Bones of the thorax

The thoracic cavity contains organs such as the heart and lungs, which are protected by the rib cage.

③ **Ribs** – there are 12 pairs of ribs.

④ **Sternum** – also known as the breast bone.

Bones of the upper limbs

⑤ **Humerus** – the long bone of the upper arm.

Bones of the vertebral column (spine)

The vertebral column supports the upper body and encloses and protects the spinal cord. It consists of 33 bones, which are divided into five groups – **cervical, thoracic, lumbar, sacral** and **coccygeal**.

The ① **cervical spine** consists of seven vertebrae.

The ② **thoracic spine** consists of 12 vertebrae.

The ③ **lumbar spine** consists of five bones, which are the largest vertebrae.

The ④ **sacrum** consists of five vertebrae fused together.

The ⑤ **coccyx** consists of four bones fused together.

= 33 bones.

Intervertebral discs

In between the bones of the spine are pads of white fibrocartilage known as intervertebral discs. The intervertebral discs are thicker in the lumbar region than in the cervical region and are kept in place by ligaments. Their functions are to act as shock absorbers and to give the spine some flexibility so movement can be made.

ARTHRITIS

The term 'arthritis' refers to many different diseases, most of which are characterised by inflammation of one or more joints. Pain and stiffness may also be present in muscles near the joint. The two main kinds are rheumatoid arthritis and ostoarthritis. Rheumatoid is the most severe form of arthritis and will affect one person in 100. Osteoarthritis is the most common form of arthritis and will affect one in 10.

Task 2.19

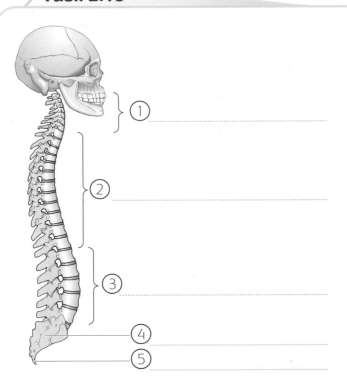

① ....

② ....

③ ....

④ ....

⑤ ....

Figure 2.8   *Bones of the vertebral column*

Label the diagrams in Figure 2.8, using the information on page 53.

Note

The **atlas** is the first cervical vertebra and consists of a ring of bone. Below it is the second cervical vertebra, called the **axis**, the shape of which allows the top of it to sit inside the atlas. The joining of these bones allows the side-to-side movement of the head.

The muscular system

There are over 600 muscles in the body, which make up 40–50% of the body weight. The function of the muscles is to produce movement, maintain posture and provide heat for the body.

The muscular system consists of three types of muscle, **involuntary**, **cardiac** and **voluntary**.

Involuntary muscle is also known as **smooth muscle**. Such muscles are involuntary because they are not under our conscious control. The cells of the muscles are spindle-shaped. Smooth muscle makes up the walls of tubular organs, e.g. the alimentary canal. It is also found in the walls of blood and lymph vessels. The muscles allow the walls to relax and constrict.

The **cardiac muscle** is specialised tissue found only in the heart. This muscle never tires; if it did we would have serious problems! Even if the heart is separated from the body, it will continue to beat for a while.

Therapists are mostly concerned with **voluntary muscles**, which are under our conscious control and are also known as the **skeletal muscles**.

Skeletal muscles consist of bundles of muscle fibres, striped in appearance and enclosed in a sheath (fascia). They allow movement of the body (Figure 2.9).

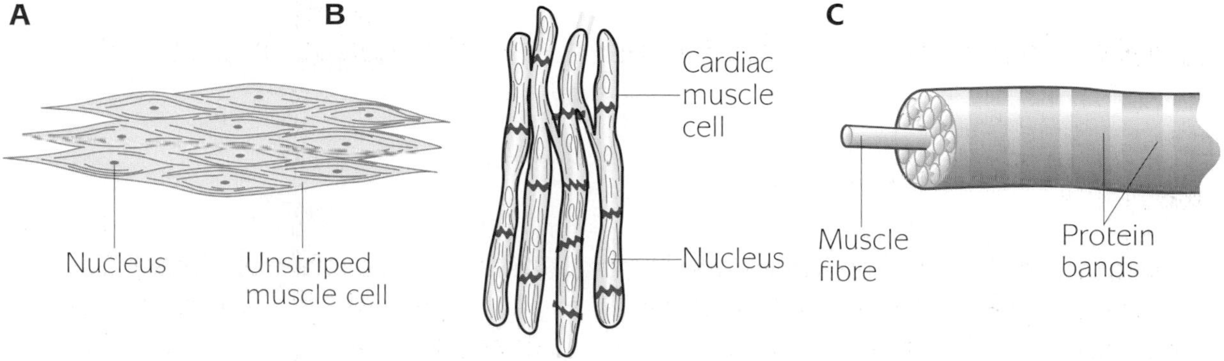

Note

There are over 600 muscles in the body.

A

B

C

Nucleus

Unstriped muscle cell

Cardiac muscle cell

Nucleus

Muscle fibre

Protein bands

Figure 2.9 *Types of muscle:* **A** *involuntary (smooth) muscle;* **B** *cardiac muscle;* **C** *voluntary (skeletal) muscle*

THE ACTION OF MUSCLES

Muscle contraction

Skeletal muscle tissue consists of bundles of long, thin muscle fibres. Inside each fibre are thread-like **myofibrils,** which extend the entire length of the muscle fibre. Myofibrils contain two types of overlapping protein called filaments, which lie side by side. They do not extend the whole length of the muscle fibre but are arranged into sections. The thinner filaments are called **actin,** and the thicker filaments are known as **myosin.** The overlapping of these filaments gives muscle fibres their striped appearance. When a muscle contracts, it shortens and thickens. This is because the thinner filaments (actin) slide in between the thicker filaments (myosin). When the muscle relaxes the thinner filaments slide back out again (Figures 2.10 and 2.11).

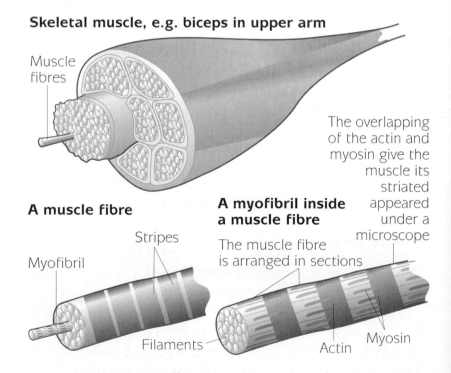

Skeletal muscle, e.g. biceps in upper arm

Muscle fibres

The overlapping of the actin and myosin give the muscle its striated appeared under a microscope

A muscle fibre

Myofibril

Stripes

Filaments

A myofibril inside a muscle fibre

The muscle fibre is arranged in sections

Actin

Myosin

Figure 2.10   *The interior of a muscle*

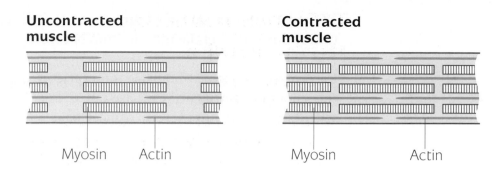

Figure 2.11 *The mechanism of contraction of a muscle*

Skeletal muscles are richly supplied with blood vessels and nerves. Before movement of a muscle can occur a message must be sent from the brain through a motor nerve, which will in turn stimulate the muscle to contract. The point at which a motor nerve enters a muscle is called the **motor point**. A motor nerve branches out, the ends of which are called **motor end plates** and rest on muscle fibres. Each muscle fibre has its own nerve ending. Branches of one motor nerve can stimulate up to 150 muscle fibres at any one time.

The bundles of muscle fibres are covered in fibrous tissue, also called **fascia**. This tissue extends to become **tendons** and attaches the muscle to bone.

Skeletal muscles bring about movement by exerting a pull on tendons, which cause the bones to move at the joints. The pulling force that causes movement is due to contraction (shortening) of the muscle.

Muscle tone

Muscle is never completely at rest but in a state of partial contraction. The partial contraction is not enough to move the muscle but will cause some tension. All skeletal muscles must be slightly contracted if the body is to remain upright. If all of the muscles relaxed then the body would fall to the floor. This continuous slight tension is involuntary and is known as **muscle tone**.

Different groups of muscle fibres contract at different times; this prevents the muscle from becoming fatigued.

Each person's degree of muscle tone varies depending on the amount of activity or exercise taken. People who are sedentary and do not exercise usually have poor muscle tone as the muscle fibres do not contract as far as they should. This results in a lowering of muscle tone and so the muscles are said to be **flaccid**. Muscles with a high degree of tone are called **spastic** as they are hard and rigid as a result of over-contraction. This can be seen in body-builders. Regular exercise and massage can help to maintain the elasticity of the of muscle fibres, which will improve the tone of the muscle.

Muscle fatigue

Muscles require fuel in the form of glucose, and oxygen is needed to burn the glucose to release energy. When muscles become overworked, such as happens during vigorous exercise, the oxygen and glucose supplies are used up. If there is insufficient oxygen and glucose the muscles cannot produce enough energy to contract. The contractions will be become weaker until they eventually stop. This is known as **muscle fatigue**.

As a result, an accumulation of harmful waste products such as lactic acid and carbon dioxide starts to build up in the affected muscle, causing stiffness and pain. Muscle fatigue is common among athletes who compete in endurance sports such as marathon races. Resting and gentle massage of the muscle will ensure that the blood brings oxygen and glucose and removes the waste products so that the muscles can work properly again.

Muscle strain

Overwork or overstretching of the muscles can cause strain and may result in muscle fibres being torn. It can normally be felt as hardness in the muscle, usually running the same way as the muscle fibres.

> **Note**
>
> Poor diet or lack of use can cause muscles to atrophy (waste away).

> **Note**
>
> A build-up of lactic acid can also cause a condition called 'fibrositis', in which there is stiffness, pain and inflammation in the affected muscle.

Tearing of muscle fibres

Injury to a muscle can cause complete or partial tearing of the muscle fibres. Partial tears result in the tearing of some muscle fibres and will feel very tender and painful, especially when contracting the muscle. Complete tearing involves tearing of all the muscle fibres, which causes the two ends of the muscle to contract away from each other. It is extremely painful and there is complete loss of function.

Cramp

Cramp is a painful muscle spasm that may arise following exercise. Muscle spasms occur when muscles contract for too long, or when excessive sweating causes water and salt loss. The accumulation of lactic acid in the muscles following vigorous exercise may also cause cramp. Lightly massaging and gradually stretching the affected muscle can relieve the spasm and pain. Sometimes cramp can occur for no reason, for example during sleep, and may be due to poor muscle tone.

Effects of temperature

Exercise is an effective way of increasing body temperature because when muscles are working they produce heat. When muscle tissue is warm the muscle fibres contract more easily as the blood circulation is increased. Therefore the chemical reactions that naturally take place in the muscle cells are speeded up. When muscle tissue is cold the opposite happens: the chemical reactions slow down and so contraction will be slower.

EFFECTS OF MASSAGE ON MUSCLES

⬧ The blood supply to the muscle is increased during massage bringing fresh oxygen and nutrients and removing waste products such as lactic acid, so massage can help to alleviate muscle fatigue. The muscle is warmed because of the increased blood flow and, because warm muscles contract more efficiently than when cold, the likelihood of injury is reduced.

Note

Vigorous exercise can cause minor tearing of muscle fibres and is thought to be a major reason why muscles become sore and stiff 12–48 hours afterwards.

- Massage helps to relieve pain, stiffness and fatigue in muscles as the waste products are removed and normal functioning is quickly restored. The increased oxygen and nutrients aid tissue repair and recovery of the muscle.

- Massage can help the breakdown of fibrositic nodules, also termed knots, that develop within a muscle because of tension, injuries or poor posture. They are commonly found in the shoulder area.

- Massage helps to increase the tone of the muscles and delays wasting away of muscles through lack of use.

Task 2.20

Fill in the gaps in the following text.
- There are over _____ muscles in the body.
- The three types of muscle are _____, _____ and _____.
- Skeletal muscles are an example of _____ muscles.
- When a muscle contracts the thinner filaments, _____, slide in between the thicker filaments, called _____.
- A _____ nerve stimulates the muscle to contract.
- Muscle _____ is the slight tension in which the muscles are continually held.
- When there is a low degree of muscle tone, the muscles are said to be _____.
- When there is a high degree of muscle tone, the muscles are said to be _____.
- Muscle fatigue occurs when there is insufficient _____ and _____.
- Stiffness and pain results when the waste products _____ _____ and _____ _____ accumulate in the muscle.
- Injury to a muscle can cause complete or partial _____ of the muscle fibres.
- Fibrositic nodules can develop as a result of _____, _____ or _____ _____.

MUSCLES OF THE BODY

Table 2.1   Muscles of the head, face and neck

Muscle	Position	Action
① **Frontalis**	Across the forehead	Draws scalp forward and raises eyebrows
② **Corrugator**	Between the eyebrows	Lowers eyebrows and wrinkles skin of forehead, as in frowning
③ **Buccinator**	In each cheek, to the side of the mouth	Compresses cheeks, as in whistling and blowing, and draws the corners of the mouth in, as in sucking
④ **Risorius**	Extends diagonally from either side of the mouth	Draws the corner of the mouth outwards, as in grinning
⑤ **Masseter**	The cheeks	The muscle of chewing: it closes the mouth and clenches the teeth
⑥ **Orbicularis oculi**	Around the eyes	Closes the eye
⑦ **Zygomaticus major**	Extends diagonally from the corners of the mouth	Lifts the corners of the mouth upwards and outwards, as in smiling or laughing
⑧ **Mentalis**	On the chin	Raises and protrudes lower lip, wrinkles skin of chin
⑨ **Orbicularis oris**	Surrounds the mouth	Closure and protrusion of the lips, changes shape of lips for speech
⑩ **Temporalis**	Extends from the temple region to the upper jaw bone	Raises the lower jaw and draws it backwards, as in chewing
⑪ **Sterno-cleidomastoid**	Runs from the top of the sternum to the clavicle and temporal bones	Both together bend head forward; one muscle only rotates the head and draws it towards the opposite shoulder
⑫ **Platysma**	Extends from the lower jaw to the chest and covers the front of the neck	Depresses lower jaw and draws lower lip outwards and draws up the skin of the chest
⑬ **Levator anguli oris**	On the cheek	Raises the corner of the mouth, as in smiling
⑭ **Levator labii superioris**	On the cheek	Lifts the upper lip, as in smiling
⑮ **Depressor anguli oris**	On the chin	Draws the corners of the mouth down, as in frowning
⑯ **Depressor labii inferioris**	On the chin	Lowers the bottom lip

Table 2.1 (continued)

⑰	**Nasalis**	Sides of the nose	Opens the nostrils, as when angry
⑱	**Procerus**	On the nasal bone	Causes the small horizontal lines between the eyebrows when angry
⑲	**Occipitalis**	At the back of the head	Draws the scalp backwards
⑳	**Pterygoids (lateral and medial)**	Outer part of the cheek	Moves the mandible from side to side, as in chewing
㉑	**Triangularis**	Chin	Lowers the corners of the mouth
㉒	**Splenius capitis**	Back of the neck	These muscles work together to move the head to an upright position

Note

The **frontalis** is joined to the **occipitalis** muscle by a strong, flat, broad tendon called the **epicranial aponeurosis**, which acts as a hat, covering the scalp.

Note

Superficial muscles are found nearer the surface of the body. **Deep** muscles are found deeper inside the body.

Origin and insertion

The **origin** of a muscle is the bone to which it is attached that does not move. The **insertion** is the bone to which the muscle is attached that does move. For example, the biceps of the upper arm has its point of origin at the shoulder, while the point of insertion is the radius of the lower arm. The insertion is the part farthest away from the spine. Muscles always move towards their origins.

Muscles in the body normally work in pairs to produce movement. During movement one muscle will contract while another relaxes.

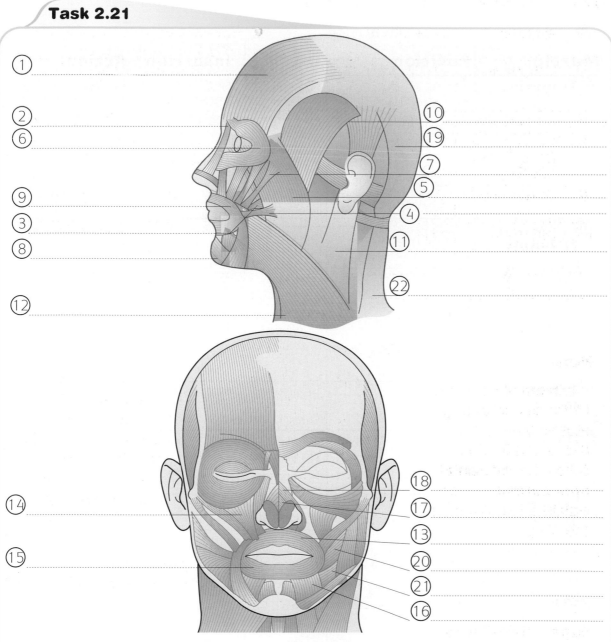

Figure 2.12 *Muscles of the face and neck*

Label the diagrams in Figure 2.12, using the information in Table 2.1.

Table 2.2   Muscles of the shoulders and back

Muscle	Position	Origin	Insertion	Action
① **Trapezius**	Forms a large, kite-shaped muscle across the top of the back and neck	Occipital bone and vertebrae	Scapula and clavicle	Lifts the clavicle, as in shrugging and also draws the head backwards
② **Deltoid**	A thick, triangular muscle that caps the shoulder	Clavicle and scapula	Humerus	Abducts the arm and draws it backwards and forwards
③ **Infra-spinatus**	Deep muscle that covers the lower part of the scapula	Scapula	Humerus	Outwardly rotates and adducts arm
④ **Supra-spinatus**	Deep muscle that covers the upper part of the scapula	Scapula	Humerus	Helps deltoid muscle to abduct arm
⑤ **Teres major**	Deep muscle across back of shoulders	Scapula	Humerus	Helps to inwardly rotate and adduct arm
⑥ **Teres minor**	Deep muscle across back of shoulders	Scapula	Humerus	Outwardly rotates and adducts arm
⑦ **Rhomboids**	Between vertebral column and scapula	Thoracic vertebrae	Scapula	Rotate and adduct (pull) scapula towards spine
⑧ **Levator scapulae**	At back and side of neck, on to scapula	Cervical vertebrae	Scapula	Lifts shoulder and scapula
⑨ **Coracobrachialis**	Upper part of arm, beneath deltoid	Scapula	Humerus	Flexes and adducts arm
⑩ **Erector spinae**	Three groups of muscles found on either side of vertebrae	Vertebrae, ribs, iliac crest	Cervical and lumbar vertebrae, ribs	Extends the spine and so helps to hold the body in an upright position
⑪ **Latissimus dorsi**	A large sheet of muscle down the back of the lower thorax and lumbar region	Vertebrae	Humerus	Draws the arm back and inwards towards the body; helps to pull body upwards when climbing

Back of body

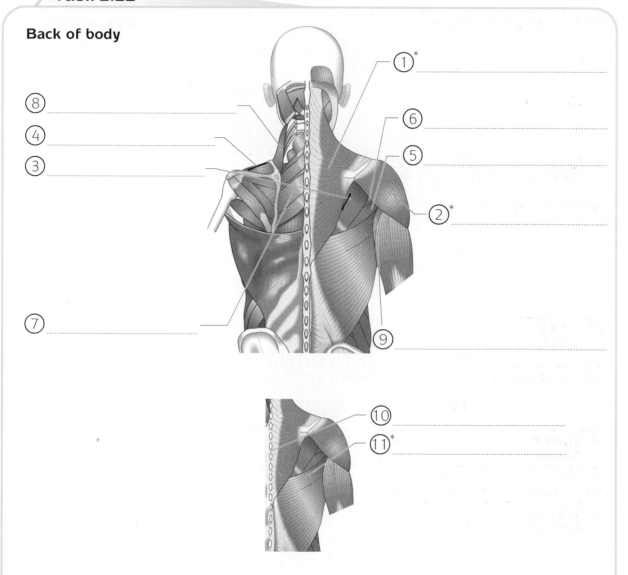

Figure 2.13 *Muscles of the shoulders and back.*
★ These are the muscles you will be working directly over when massaging.
The other muscles are deeper.

Label the diagram in Figure 2.13, using the information in Table 2.2.

Muscles of the upper limbs

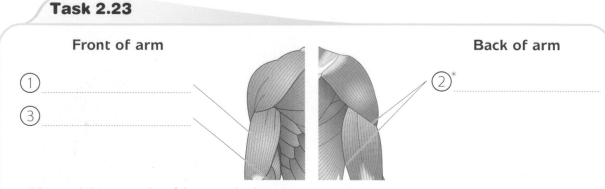

Front of arm

① ....

③ ....

Back of arm

②* ....

Figure 2.14 *Muscles of the upper limb*

Label the diagram in Figure 2.14, using the information in Table 2.3.
*This muscle is superficial, so you will be working directly over it when massaging.

Table 2.3   **Muscles of the upper limbs**

Muscle	Position	Origin	Insertion	Action
① **Biceps brachii**	Down anterior surface of the humerus	Scapula	Radius and flexor muscles in forearm	Flexes the forearm
② **Triceps**	Posterior surface of the humerus	Humerus and scapula	Ulna	Extends the forearm
③ **Brachialis**	On the anterior aspect of humerus beneath the biceps	Humerus	Ulna	Flexes the forearm

Note

Adduction means movement of body part towards midline of body.
Abduction means movement of body part away from midline of body.

Muscles of the chest

① ....

② ....

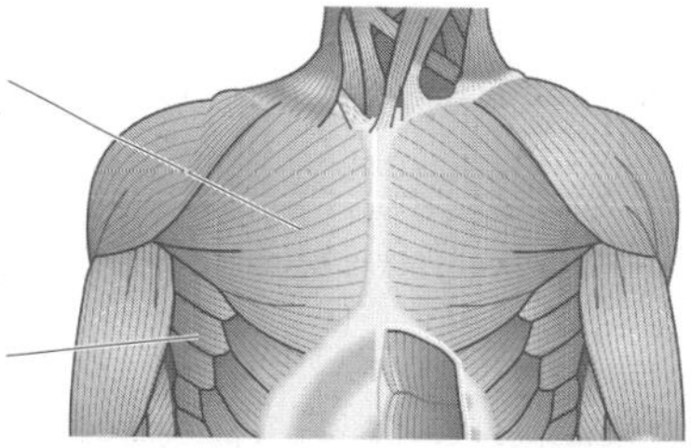

Figure 2.15   *Muscles of the chest*

Label the diagram in Figure 2.15, using the information in Table 2.4.

Table 2.4   **Muscles of the chest**

Muscle	Position	Origin	Insertion	Action
① **Pectoralis major**	Covers the upper part of the thorax clavicle	Sternum, ribs and	Humerus	Adducts and inwardly rotates the arm
② **Serratus anterior**	Sides of the ribcage below the armpits	Ribs	Scapula	Draws scapula forward, as in pushing movements

Note

Flexion is the bending of a body part.
Extension means straightening of a body part.

POSTURE

A good posture means that the body is aligned and balanced, so that the work carried out by muscles to maintain it is kept to a minimum. It will ensure that muscles and joints are working efficiently so that the body remains free from muscular tension, strains, stiffness and pain. A poor posture means that the body is out of balance so that certain muscles have to contract strongly to maintain it. Over a period of time these muscles will tighten and shorten, while others will stretch and weaken. Three main postural faults are lordosis, kyphosis and scoliosis (Figure 2.16).

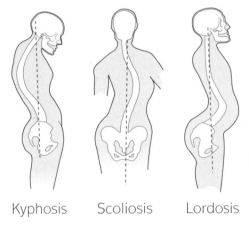

Kyphosis   Scoliosis   Lordosis

Figure 2.16   *Postural faults*

Lordosis

Lordosis is a condition that shows itself as an inward exaggeration of the lumbar region of the spine. The client will appear to have a hollow back and there will be protrusion of the abdomen and buttocks. Gymnasts often adopt this posture.

Kyphosis

Kyphosis is a condition where there is an exaggeration of the thoracic curve of the spine. The client will have rounded shoulders and the chin pokes forwards.

Adopting a poor posture often causes kyphosis.

Note

In kyphosis the upper back muscles are weakened and overstretched. The pectoral muscles are tightened and shortened.

Scoliosis

A feature of scoliosis is a lateral curvature of the spine, which may be C or S shaped. It can result in the level of the shoulders and pelvic girdle being slightly uneven. An individual may be born with this condition or the continual carrying of heavy bags on one particular shoulder over a period of time can cause it. The muscles that are shortened are found on the inside of the curve and the muscles that are overstretched are found on the outside of the curve. Shortened and tight muscles can be relaxed and stretched with massage so helping to correct posture faults.

Blood circulation

The cardiovascular system consists of the heart, blood and blood vessels. The function of the heart is to act as a pump to move the blood around the body. The blood carries oxygen and nutrients and is transported in the body by blood vessels.

BLOOD PLASMA

Plasma is the liquid part of the blood and mainly consists of water. Many substances can travel in the blood plasma, including blood cells, hormones, nutrients and the waste products produced by cells.

FUNCTIONS OF THE BLOOD

The functions of the blood include:

- **Delivers** oxygen, nutrients and hormones to the cells of the body. Heat is also transported around the body from the muscles and liver, which helps regulate the body temperature.
- **Removes** carbon dioxide and waste from the cells.

> **Note**
>
> To help you remember the functions of the blood think of: **D-R-A-C**-ula.
>
> **D** – delivers
>
> **R** – removes
>
> **A** – attacks
>
> **C** – clots.

- **Attacks** harmful organisms such as bacteria. The white blood cells protect the body against disease.
- **Clots** the blood to prevents excess loss of blood if an injury should occur to the body.

BLOOD CELLS

Red blood cells

Red blood cells (erythrocytes) are button-shaped cells that are made in the bone marrow and live for about 3 months (Figure 2.17). There are approximately 5 million of these cells in a drop of blood. Red blood cells contain the pigment **haemoglobin**. The oxygen picked up from the lungs combines with the haemoglobin. The function of red blood cells is to carry oxygen around the body and deliver it to the cells. The cells use the oxygen and nutrients and produce carbon dioxide. Carbon dioxide can be carried away by the red blood cells and taken back to the lungs to be breathed out.

Haemoglobin is rich in iron and needs a constant supply. Iron comes from the food we eat and also from old or damaged red blood cells that have been destroyed by the liver.

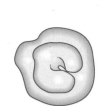
Leucocyte
(white blood cell)

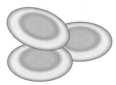
Erythrocytes
(red blood cells)

Thrombocytes
(platelets)

Figure 2.17 *Blood cells*

White blood cells

White blood cells (leucocytes) contain a nucleus and are larger than red blood cells. There are up to 10 000 in a drop of blood. Most types of white blood cell can change their shape so they are able to squeeze through small spaces. Therefore, white blood cells are able to reach almost anywhere in the body. The function of white blood cells is to protect us from disease.

All blood cells are made in the bone marrow. Of the white cells, 75% go directly into circulation and the other 25% are processed in the lymphatic system to gain specialist methods of combat against infection. These cells are called **granulocytes** because they have tiny granules in their cytoplasm. Most granulocytes are **phagocytes** – this means that they are able to engulf and digest (eat) bacteria and any other harmful matter.

Agranulocytes do not have granules in their cytoplasm. These white cells make up the remaining 25% and are mostly produced in the lymphatic system. Lymphocytes and monocytes are types of agranulocyte.

The job of **lymphocytes** is to produce **antibodies**. Antibodies are chemicals made by the body in response to bacteria and any other harmful matter. They have the function of destroying harmful matter so that it is no longer a threat to the body.

Monocytes destroy harmful matter, e.g. bacteria, by engulfing and digesting them, like most of the granulocytes. These cells gather around wounds and kill invading bacteria to prevent them from entering the body.

Note

Leukaemia is a cancer caused by the overproduction of white blood cells.

Platelets

Platelets (thrombocytes) are tiny fragments of cells, which are smaller than white and red blood cells. They are produced in the bone marrow and live for up to 2 weeks. There are about 200 000 in a drop of blood. Platelets are involved with the clotting process of the blood following an injury to the body. Their function is to help to prevent loss of blood from damaged blood vessels by forming a plug.

Blood is transported around the body in a series of pipes called blood vessels (Figure 2.19). These blood vessels are called arteries, arterioles, capillaries, venules and veins, and form an intricate network within the body.

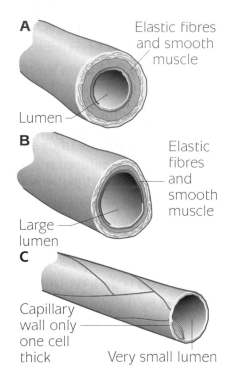

Figure 2.19 *Blood vessels:* **A** *artery;* **B** *vein;* **C** *capillary*

Arteries

Arteries have thick, elastic, muscular walls because the blood within them is carried under high pressure, because of the pumping action of the heart. Arteries carry blood **away from** the heart. All arteries carry **oxygenated** blood, with the exception of the pulmonary arteries, which carry deoxygenated blood from the heart to the lungs. Arteries are generally deep-seated, except where they cross a pulse spot, such as the radial artery in the wrist and carotid artery in the neck where a pulse can be felt. As arteries get further from the heart they branch off and become smaller. The oxygenated blood eventually reaches very small arteries called **arterioles**.

Capillaries

Arterioles are connected to the capillaries. Capillaries are the smallest vessels, about a hundredth of a millimetre thick. Unlike arteries and veins, the walls of the capillaries are thin enough to allow certain substances to pass through them – this is known as **capillary exchange**. Oxygen and nutrients are delivered to the cells of the body and carbon dioxide and waste products are removed.

The capillaries connect with larger vessels called **venules**. Now that oxygen has been removed from the blood and carbon dioxide has been picked up, by the time the blood reaches the venules it has become deoxygenated (Figure 2.20).

Note

Capillaries are so small that the red blood cells have to pass through in single file.

Note

There are over 60 000 miles of capillaries in the body.

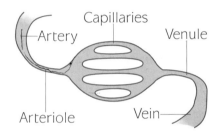

Figure 2.20 *How blood passes from arteries through capillaries to veins*

Veins

Blood flows through the venules until it reaches larger vessels called veins. The veins carry blood, called venous blood, **towards** the heart. Their walls are thinner and less elastic than arteries. Veins carry **deoxygenated** blood, with the exception of the pulmonary veins, which carry oxygenated blood from the lungs to the heart. Veins are nearer the surface of the body than the arteries. Unlike the other blood vessels, veins contain **valves**, which prevent the blood from flowing backwards (Figure 2.21).

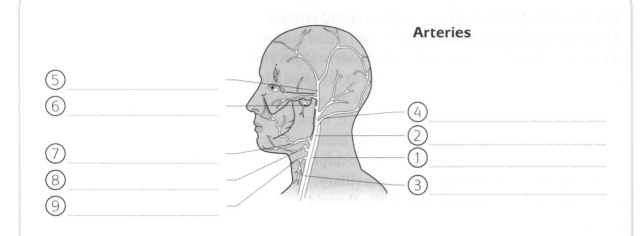

Arteries

⑤ ....

⑥ ....

⑦ ....

⑧ ....

⑨ ....

④ ....

② ....

① ....

③ ....

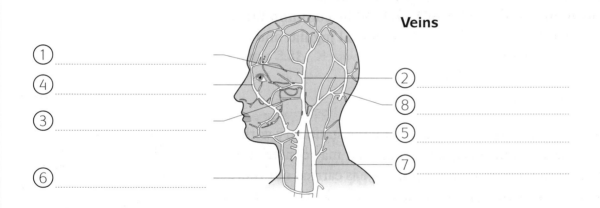

Veins

① ....

④ ....

③ ....

⑥ ....

② ....

⑧ ....

⑤ ....

⑦ ....

Figure 2.22 *Blood vessels of the head and neck:* **A** *arteries;* **B** *veins*

Label the diagram in Figure 2.22, using the information on page 77.

Blood pressure

When blood reaches the capillaries it is vital that oxygen and nutrients pass out of the blood and into the cells. It is the pressure of blood that forces fluid out through the capillary walls. The fluid contains oxygen and nutrients that pass into the cell by diffusion. Therefore, it is important for the body to maintain the correct level of blood pressure.

High/low blood pressure

High blood pressure (hypertension) is when the blood pressure is consistently above normal. It can lead to strokes and heart attacks as the heart has to work harder to force blood through the system. High blood pressure can be caused by smoking, obesity, lack of exercise, eating too much salt, stress, too much alcohol, the contraceptive pill, pregnancy and hereditary factors. Massage and certain essential oils can be beneficial for people suffering with this condition but a doctor's permission should be sought prior to treatment.

Low blood pressure (hypotension) is when the blood pressure is below normal for a substantial time. Blood pressure must be sufficient to pump blood to the brain when the body is in the upright position. If it is not then the person will feel faint. Some people with low blood pressure may feel faint when sitting up suddenly from the lying position.

EFFECTS OF MASSAGE ON THE BLOOD CIRCULATORY SYSTEM

Massage causes the blood vessels to be compressed, forcing blood forward. As pressure is released the blood vessels return to their normal size and blood rushes in to fill the space created. Reddening of the skin, called erythema, results. Fresh, oxygenated blood and nutrients are brought to the area and so will nourish the tissues and help with tissue repair. Waste products (metabolic waste) are removed and carried away by the veins. A build-up of waste products can cause pain and stiffness and so massage can help to relieve these symptoms.

Massage movements such as effleurage (stroking) will help to return the blood in the veins back to the heart (venous return). This is why strokes are performed in the direction of the venous flow.

The lymphatic system

Have you noticed that certain glands swell up when you are ill, such as the glands in the neck, which inflame during a throat infection? The glands you can feel are lymph nodes. Lymph nodes, lymph, lymph vessels and lymphatic ducts all make up the lymphatic system, which is closely related to the blood circulation.

HOW IS LYMPH DERIVED?

Blood does not flow into the tissues but remains inside the blood vessels. However, plasma from the blood is able to seep through the capillary walls and enter the spaces between the tissues. This fluid provides the cells with nutrients and oxygen. It has now become tissue fluid, also known as **interstitial fluid**. More fluid passes out of the blood capillaries than is returned to the blood. The excess tissue fluid passes into the lymphatic capillaries and now becomes **lymph**. Lymph is similar to blood plasma but contains more white blood cells (Figure 2.23 opposite).

THE FUNCTIONS OF THE LYMPHATIC SYSTEM

- **Helps to fight infection** – the production of lymphocytes and antibodies by the lymphatic system is

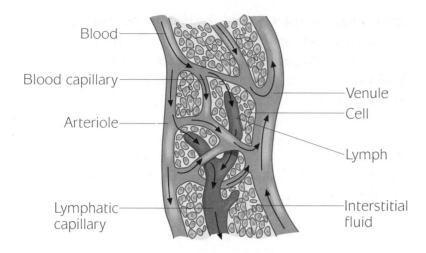

Figure 2.23 *The relationship between blood and lymph*

Labels: Blood, Blood capillary, Arteriole, Lymphatic capillary, Venule, Cell, Lymph, Interstitial fluid

an important part of the immune system. Lymphocytes (white blood cells) recognise harmful substances and destroy them.

- **Distributes fluid in the body** – lymphatic vessels drain approximately 3 litres of excess tissue fluid daily from tissue spaces.

- **Transport of fats** – carbohydrates and protein are passed from the small intestine directly into the bloodstream. However, fats are passed from the small intestine into lymphatic vessels called lacteals before eventually passing into the bloodstream. It is uncertain why fats are absorbed via the lymphatic system.

LYMPH NODES

There are approximately 600 bean-shaped lymph nodes scattered throughout the body. They lie mainly in groups around the groin, breast, armpits and round the major blood vessels of the abdomen and chest.

Lymph is a watery, colourless fluid that passes through the lymph nodes. Lymph nodes filter out harmful substances from the lymph, such as bacteria, which could cause an infection in the body. They contain specialised white blood cells called lymphocytes and monocytes. Monocytes destroy harmful substances by ingesting (eating) them; lymphocytes produce antibodies that stop the growth of bacteria and prevent their harmful action. During an infection there are more bacteria and so the lymph nodes produce more lymphocytes to destroy them. This causes the lymph nodes to enlarge and is a sign that the glands are working to fight the infection.

Task 2.27

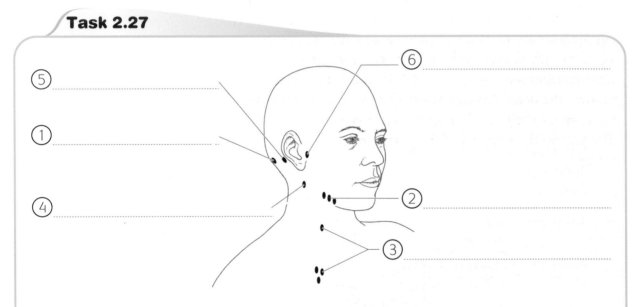

Figure 2.24   *Lymph glands of the head and neck*

Label the diagram in Figure 2.24, using the information below.

Important groups of lymph nodes in the head are the ① **occipital**, ② **submandibular**, ③ **deep cervical**, ④ **superficial cervical**, ⑤ **posterior auricular** and ⑥ **anterior auricular** glands.

LYMPH VESSELS

Lymph travels around the body in one direction only, towards the heart. It is carried in vessels that begin as lymphatic capillaries. Lymph capillaries are blind-ended tubes, situated between cells, and are found throughout the body. The walls of lymphatic capillaries are structured in such a way that tissue fluid can pass into them but not out of them.

Lymphatic capillaries join up and become wider tubes, known as lymphatic vessels. The lymph vessels generally run parallel to the veins. These vessels are similar to veins as they contain valves, although they generally have thinner walls (Figure 2.25). The lymph flows around the body through these lymph vessels and passes through a number of lymph nodes to be filtered. Eventually the lymph will be passed into lymphatic ducts.

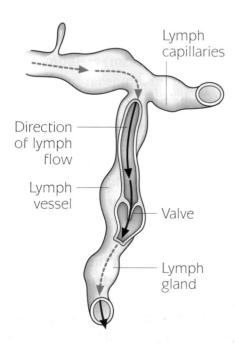

Figure 2.25 *The flow of lymph through a lymphatic vessel*

Note

Bell's palsy is a condition in which one side of the face becomes paralysed, so that it drops. It can be due to a viral infection or an injury of the facial nerves. Facial massage may help to prevent wasting of the affected facial muscles.

The fifth cranial nerve, called the **trigeminal nerve**, is the largest. This nerve sends messages to the brain from sensory nerves in the face, teeth and part of the scalp. It has three branches: the **ophthalmic nerve** ①, the **maxillary nerve** ② and the **mandibular nerve** ③.

The seventh cranial nerve (the **facial nerve**), passes through the temporal bone to behind the ear. It supplies the tongue, palate and muscles of the face. Branches from this nerve include ④ **cervical nerves** and ⑤ **buccal nerves**.

Other nerves that supply the head, neck and shoulders include the ⑥ **frontal nerves**, ⑦ **lacrimal nerves**, ⑧ **infraorbital nerves**, ⑨ **lingual nerves** and ⑩ **supraclavicular nerves**.

Task 2.29

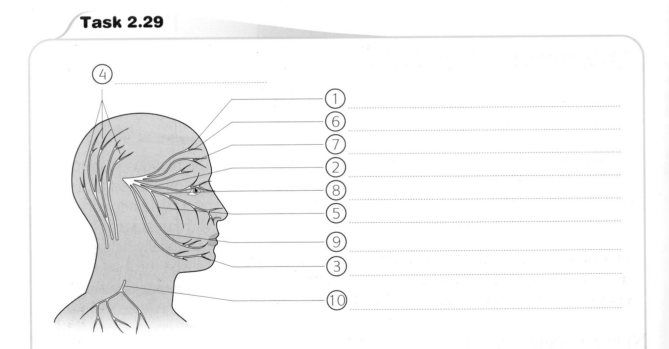

Figure 2.27 *Important nerves of the head*

Label the diagram in Figure 2.27, using the information above.

The olfactory system

Note

A professional perfumier can distinguish 100 000 different odours.

The olfactory system provides us with the sense of smell, also known as olfaction. The brain is able to distinguish about 20 000 different scents, with the help of the nervous system. Millions of olfactory receptors in the nose transmit messages in the form of nerve impulses to the brain.

HOW IS SMELL PERCEIVED?

Substances such as essential oils (oils used in aromatherapy) give off ① **smelly gas particles**. These particles are drawn into the nose as we inhale and dissolve into the upper part of the moist mucous membrane of the nasal cavity.

The ② **mucus** surrounds small hairs called ③ **cilia** that stick out from the bottom of ④ **olfactory cells**. The gas particles reach the cilia and stimulate nerve impulses to travel along the ⑤ **axon of the nerve cell**, through bones in the skull and to the ⑥ **olfactory bulb**, of which there are two.

Nerves from the olfactory bulb then carry nerve impulses to the brain. The ⑦ **limbic system** in the brain interprets the information received from the olfactory bulbs as smell, and we become aware of it.

The limbic system also deals with emotions such as pain, anger, pleasure, affection and memory. This is why smells can evoke different emotional responses and can bring back a flood of memories.

ADAPTION

We can become adapted to a smell. If we spray perfume we will soon stop noticing its smell because the olfactory receptors, of which there are millions, will stop being stimulated until a new smell comes along.

Note

Ensure that you also send a leaflet briefly explaining the treatment, as the doctor may not know what an Indian head massage is!

from their doctor regarding their medical condition and their suitability for treatment. It is a good idea to have a standard letter, which a client can give to the doctor or post enclosing a stamped, addressed envelope. The doctor need only sign his/her name to advise the patient that there is a medical reason why treatment should not go ahead. A sample letter is illustrated in Figure 3.2.

Doctors do not often know what an Indian head massage treatment entails and therefore cannot give permission as such for treatment to go ahead, only tell their patient whether or not they think it is advisable. A doctor's insurance does not cover them for giving permission or consent to holistic therapy treatments.

Address of treatment room

Date

Dr's address

Dear Dr *(name)*
Your patient, *(name)* of *(his/her address)*, has informed me that he/she is suffering with *(high blood pressure, diabetes, etc.)*.

Please tell me if in your view there is any reason why your patient should not have Indian head massage treatment.

Thank you.

Yours sincerely,

(Your signature)

(Your name printed)

Doctor's advice
I feel that *(name of client)* would/would not be suuitable for Indian head massage treatment.

Doctor's signature ______________________ Date __________

Figure 3.2 *A sample advice letter to a client's GP*

HANDLING REFERRAL DATA FROM PROFESSIONAL SOURCES

If a healthcare professional, whether a doctor or a reflexologist, etc., refers a client to you for Indian head massage treatment, it is courteous to keep them informed of the client's progress. A progress report should include the following information:

- the client's name, who referred them and their reason for coming for Indian head massage treatment
- the client's progress
- treatment plan for the future.

A brief letter can be written reporting the progress of a client, an example of which is given in Figure 3.3.

Note

Why not write to your client's husband or wife a couple of weeks before your client's birthday and ask if they would like to purchase a voucher from you for an Indian head massage treatment?

Note

Ensure that your client agrees to the progress report being sent.

Dr Smith
Sheldare Surgery
Bradley Stoke
Bristol

Date

Dear Dr Smith
Thank you for recommending Mrs Edwards of 11 St Peters Walk, Bradley Stoke to come to me for Indian Head Massage treatment. I am writing to inform you of her progress.

She has been having regular weekly treatments for the past month. The muscular tension has now greatly improved and there is a decrease in the number of headaches she has been suffering too.

We are to continue her treatments for two more weeks and she will then return to me on a monthly basis.

If you require further information please do not hesitate to contact me.

Yours sincerely,

Marion Willetts

Mrs M. Willets IIHHT, ITEC

Figure 3.3 *Example of a progress report to a client's GP*

PREPARING A TREATMENT PLAN

A treatment plan will ensure that you have a plan of action, which will help you and your client to reach your objectives. The plan will include the client's expectations of the treatment, thus helping to ensure client satisfaction.

Treatment plan

Client name *Mrs M. Willets*   **Date of treatment** *14th July*

Treatment given *Indian head massage*

What are the client's expectations of treatment?

* *To be relaxed*
* *To help treat the frequent headaches experienced by client*
* *To be uplifted and de-stressed*

What are the treatment objectives?

* *To help relieve muscular tension in shoulders and neck areas*
* *To prevent and treat the tension headaches frequently suffered by client*
* *To use lots of effleurage and petrissage movements and avoid too many tapotement movements to relax client*
* *To use massage movements to help lymphatic drainage, therefore draining toxins, which may be the cause of the headaches*

What oils are used, if any?

* *Sweet almond*
* *Pre-blended aromatherapy oils containing lavender and peppermint to help with muscular tension and headaches*

Any special needs?

e.g pregnancy, needs help on to the chair or perhaps specific areas need to be worked on or avoided, etc.

Recommended frequency of treatment

Weekly treatments for a period of six weeks. (This can be changed at a later date.)

Additional notes:

As the treatments progress you can add information in here such as which massage movements the client enjoys or dislikes, any problems, whether you have recommended the client to another health professional, whether the client's condition has improved or worsened, etc.

Figure 3.4 *A sample treatment plan*

At any time you can change your treatment plan to suit you and your client. You can also monitor progress to see if changes are needed in any way.

How often should a client come for treatment?

You will need to discuss with your client how often the treatment should be carried out. This will depend on their finances, the time they have available and their reasons for coming. If they have come for relaxation, perhaps they could attend once every 2 weeks; if they have a particular condition that needs treating you could advise coming for treatment once a week for 6 weeks. Emphasise to your client the importance of regular treatments to maintain the long-term benefits.

Figure 3.4 gives an example of a treatment plan.

Self-test questions

Ask yourself the following self-test questions:
1. Why is it important for the therapist to have a professional attitude towards clients?
2. Why must particular attention be paid to personal and general hygiene when treating clients?
3. What factors regarding the following should the therapist take into consideration when giving treatments?
   - Clothing
   - Hands
   - Hair
   - Jewellery
   - Shoes
4. Why is it important to be polite and greet clients with a smile?
5. Give two reasons why a therapist should wear a uniform while carrying out treatments.

6. Why is it important that the client record card is clearly written and that all the information is accurate?

7. Why is it important that all staff and clients feel safe and secure while having an Indian head massage treatment?

8. Why is it important to give accurate information to your client on the following factors?
   - The services you offer
   - Price
   - The length of time taken for treatment
   - Products sold.

9. Why is it important to establish the reasons the client has come to you and their expectations during the consultation?

10. How would you reassure a nervous client about the Indian head massage treatment?

11. Madeline suffers with regular tension headaches because of her stressful job and has problems sleeping. She often hunches at her desk so has very tense shoulders. She is expecting to be relaxed, to reduce the tension in her shoulders and to sleep well tonight. What treatment plan would you prepare for this client?

12. Why is it important to be aware of the client's body language and to react positively towards it?

13. If during the consultation your client informs you that they have a contraindication to Indian head massage, what action would you take?

Write down your answers on a sheet of paper. There are sample answers at the back of the book.

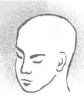
MASSAGE MOVEMENTS AND THEIR EFFECTS

While carrying out the Indian head massage routine you will use different types of massage movements called effleurage, pétrissage, tapotement, vibrations and frictions.

Effleurage

Effleurage always begins and ends the massage on each area. It is also usually performed after tapotement massage movements to soothe the area. The effleurage movement can be superficial (using light pressure) or deep, using slightly deeper pressure. These movements must always follow the direction of venous return (blood in the veins) back to the heart and also in the direction of lymphatic drainage towards a group of lymph nodes. The hands stay in contact with the body during the return stroke.

Uses of effleurage

- To distribute the massage medium so that the whole area is lubricated
- To introduce the therapist's hands
- To warm up the area so deeper massage movements can be used
- To link massage movements together, so that the massage flows
- To relax the receiver.

Note

Effleurage is a French word meaning 'stroking'.

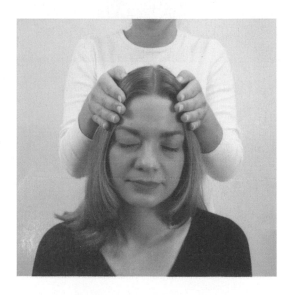

Figure 4.1 *Effleurage movement*

Effects of effleurage

◊ Improves the blood and lymphatic circulation
◊ Aids desquamation (removal of dead skin cells) so the skin will look healthier and feel smoother
◊ Soothes nerve endings, thus inducing relaxation.

Pétrissage

Pétrissage movements are deeper movements in which soft tissues are compressed. These movements either press the muscle on to the bone or lift it away from the bone. The whole hand, fingers or thumbs can be used.

There are different types of pétrissage movement:

◊ **Picking up** – The tissues are picked up and lifted away from the bone and then released. One or both hands can be used.
◊ **Kneading** – The muscle is pressed on to the bone using firm movements. This movement can be performed with the palm of one hand or both, or with the pads of the fingers or thumbs.

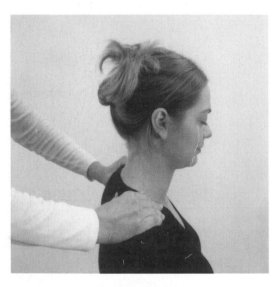

Figure 4.2 *Pétrissage movement*

Uses of pétrissage

◊ To stimulate sluggish blood circulation
◊ To aid lymphatic drainage
◊ To improve condition of skin and hair
◊ To ease muscular tension.

Effects of pétrissage

◊ Blood and lymphatic circulation is increased, encouraging the delivery of fresh oxygen and nutrients to the tissues and an increase in the rate of removal of waste products
◊ Erythema (redness) is produced
◊ The elimination of toxins is speeded up
◊ Sebum secretion is increased, thus moisturising skin and hair.

Note

Most Indian head massage movements will be a type of pétrissage.

Tapotement

Tapotement movements are also known as percussion movements. All tapotement movements are stimulating and so are usually omitted from a relaxing type of massage.

Tapotement movements include:

Note

Tapotement is a French word meaning 'drumming'.

- **Hacking,** which involves using the side of the hand, known as the ulnar border because of the bone in the forearm called the ulna. The area worked is rapidly struck using alternate hands.

- **Champi,** which is similar to hacking but the hands are placed together as in prayer. With loose wrists, the receiver's back is struck with the little-finger side of the hands.

- **Tabla playing (tapping),** which is used on the scalp and involves gently tapping on the head with your fingertips, as if playing a piano.

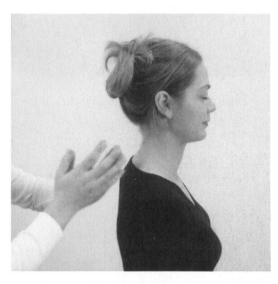

Figure 4.3 *Tapotement movement – champi*

Uses of tapotement

- To increase blood circulation to the area
- To warm the area
- To invigorate the receiver
- To tone the muscles.

Effects of tapotement

- Stimulates muscle fibres so muscle tone is improved
- Stimulates sensory nerves on either side of the spine, so it is invigorating
- Increases circulation to the area so that erythema (redness) is produced.

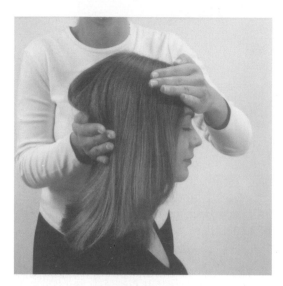

Figure 4.4 *Friction movement*

Friction

Two types of massage movement, friction and frictions, although similar in name, are completely different techniques. Friction is the fast rubbing of the skin, which is warming to it. The hands are held stiffly and the palms and fingers are used to rub quickly over the skin.

Uses of friction

◆ To increase blood supply

◆ To warm an area for further deeper work

◆ To invigorate the receiver.

Effects of friction

◆ Brings oxygen and nutrients to the area being worked

◆ Creates warmth in the area being worked.

Frictions

Frictions involve fairly deep pressure using the finger or thumb. The finger/thumb is pressed on a specific area and there is a gradual increase in pressure. A circular motion with the finger/thumb may also be used. Frictions should cause the skin to rub against structures underlying it, so that one layer of tissue is pressed firmly against another.

Uses of frictions

◆ To relieve tension in muscles, so relaxing them

◆ To increase circulation and promote healing

◆ To break down knots in muscles

◆ To stimulate and invigorate lethargic receivers.

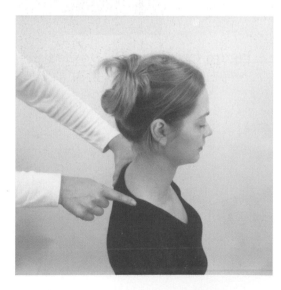

Figure 4.5 *Frictions movement*

Effects of frictions

- Stimulate the circulation, thereby bringing oxygen and nutrients to the area being worked and producing erythema
- Create warmth in area being worked
- Break down fibrous nodules (knots) in muscles
- Help to invigorate receiver when worked on either side of the spine.

Vibration

The hands or fingers of one hand are vibrated so that a fine tremor is produced in the tissues. The tremor is produced by the contraction of the forearm muscles.

Uses of vibration

- Stimulates sluggish lymphatic drainage
- Relieves tension and so induces relaxation.

Effects of vibration

- Promotes relaxation in the muscles worked as it is soothing to nerves
- Relieves pain and fatigue
- Relieves tiredness and lethargy.

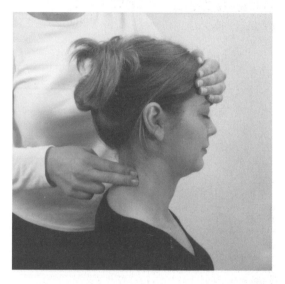

Figure 4.6 *Vibrations movement*

ADAPTING THE INDIAN HEAD MASSAGE TREATMENT

Indian head massage will sometimes have to be adapted to suit the needs of an individual.

Bald clients

An Indian head massage can be given to bald clients but certain massage movements involving the hair will obviously need to be left out. Remember not to use too much oil.

Research the uses and effects of the forms of massage movement and fill in the table below.

Movement	Two uses	Two effects
Effleurage		
Pétrissage		
Tapotement		
Friction		
Frictions		
Vibration		

Larger clients

These clients may require firmer pressure, but do consult with the client first. You may find that these clients will take a little longer to massage.

Elderly or very slim clients

These clients will probably prefer lighter pressure to be used. Care needs to be taken when massaging over bony areas as it may cause discomfort. Elderly clients can often feel the cold more easily so ensure the room is warm enough. They may need help on to the chair also.

USE OF OILS

Indian head massage treatment can be given with or without the use of oils. The main oils used in Indian head massage are sesame, mustard, olive, coconut, almond, sunflower and jojoba. The oils help to moisturise the hair and scalp, which promotes hair growth and slows down hair loss. The treatment can be carried out using vegetable oils mixed with herbs and spices.

The oils should be unrefined, as the refining process means that the oils are extracted at high temperature, resulting in nutrients being destroyed. The oils should be cold- or warm-pressed and preferably free of additives – look at the product label. With some oils it is advisable to test for allergy, particularly if the client has sensitive skin.

> **Note**
>
> If a client has come for relaxation, tapotement movements should be limited in use, as these movements are stimulating. More effleurage and stroking movements should be used instead.

Sesame oil

Sesame oil is a thick liquid with a golden yellow colour and a slight nutty aroma. Sesame seeds are extracted by shaking the dried plant upside down after making an incision in the seed pod. Sesame oil is extracted from the seeds and is the most popular oil used in India, especially in the summer months.

Sesame seeds are rich in vitamin E and minerals such as iron, calcium and phosphorus, which help nourish and protect the hair and skin.

Uses of sesame oil

- Helps to relieve muscular aches, pains and stiffness
- Moisturises dry skin and hair
- Said to prevent hair from turning grey!

Sesame oil can be used on its own or mixed with other oils such as jojoba and essential oils such as lavender. Sometimes sesame oil may irritate a sensitive skin, so an allergy test may need to be given before using it. Olive oil is an excellent alternative.

Sesame oil plays a prominent role in Indian Ayurvedic medicine. It is sometimes rubbed into the skin during abhyanga, a type of Indian massage that focuses on over 100 points on the body called marma points. Abhyanga is believed to improved energy flow and helps to free the body of impurities.

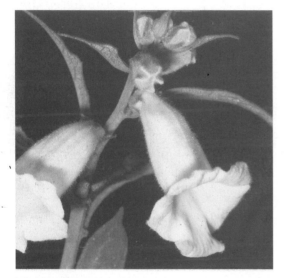

Figure 4.7 *Sesame plant* (Sesamum indicum)

Note

Sesame oil is more easily removed from clothing than most other oils.

Note

Allergy testing Place a couple of dabs of oil behind the client's ear. The oil should be left on for about 24 hours. Often, a reaction will show fairly quickly. It is advisable not to use the oil if there is redness, inflammation or itching.

Mustard oil

Mustard oil is another popular oil used in India. It is a strong-smelling, thick, yellow liquid. The oil is extracted from the crushed seeds of the mustard plant. There are large numbers of mustard plants in the north of India. Therefore, mustard oil is commonly used in this region.

Uses of mustard oil

- Relieves tension, pain and stiffness in muscles
- Encourages healthy, glossy hair growth
- Stimulates blood circulation to the scalp so helping to promote warmth; therefore, is ideal in the winter months.

Mustard oil is often used on its own because its powerful scent does not mix well with other oils. It has been known to irritate skin so an allergy test should be given before using it.

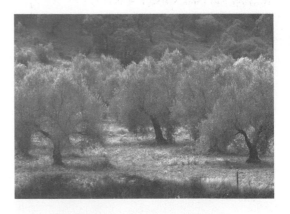

Figure 4.8 *Mustard plant* (Brassica juncaea)

Olive oil

Olive oil is a yellow-green oil extracted from the flesh of the olive. It has a thick consistency and a strong odour so is often mixed with a lighter oil such as sweet almond. It is commonly used in cooking.

Uses of olive oil

- Helps to moisturise the skin and hair so prevents dryness
- Helps to relieve muscular stiffness and pain.

It is preferable to use virgin or extra virgin oil. Olive oil is a safe oil for the skin and rarely causes irritation; it is therefore an ideal oil to use on children.

Figure 4.9 *Olive trees* (Olea europaea)

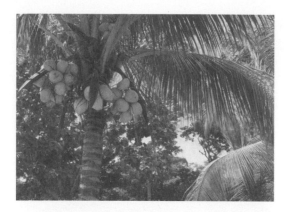

Figure 4.10 *Coconut palm (Cocos nucifera)*

Coconut oil

Coconut oil is a cream-coloured oil extracted from the dried flesh of the coconut. The oil is light and has a beautiful aroma. At room temperature coconut oil is solid but it liquefies when warmed. Placing the pot by a radiator or in warm water for a few minutes will liquefy the oil.

Coconut is highly refined, so many of the nutrients are destroyed during the refining process.

Uses of coconut oil

- Softens and moisturises the hair, so is useful for dry, brittle hair
- Encourages healthy hair growth and helps to relieve any inflammation.

Coconut oil can be used on its own or mixed with other carrier oils. It may irritate sensitive skin so an allergy test should be given. It is advisable not to use it on someone with a nut allergy.

Sweet almond oil

Sweet almond oil is extracted from the kernels of the sweet almond tree. It is a pale yellow, thick liquid that mixes well with most other carrier oils and essential oils.

It is an oil that is rich in nutrients such as unsaturated fatty acids, protein and vitamins A, B, D and E.

Uses of sweet almond oil

- Eases muscular tension, pain and stiffness
- Excellent moisturiser for skin and hair

Figure 4.11 *Sweet almond tree (Prunus dulcis)*

- Promotes healthy, glossy hair as it stimulates the blood circulation to the scalp

- Good to use on clients who have dry hair due to chemical treatments such as colouring or perms.

Sweet almond is a safe oil but it is advisable not to use it on someone suffering from a nut allergy.

Jojoba oil

Jojoba (ho-**ho**-ba) oil is a light yellow, waxy vegetable oil extracted from the crushed seeds of the jojoba plant. This evergreen shrub grows in deserts and is native to Mexico, Arizona and California. Jojoba is a nutritious oil containing vitamin E, minerals and proteins, which are absorbed into the skin. Unlike many other oils it can be heated to high temperatures and will still retain its nutrients.

At room temperature it is semisolid because of its waxy consistency but it solidifies when put in the fridge. It does not oxidise (mix with oxygen), so it keeps very well. It is good for all hair and skin types, including oily skins.

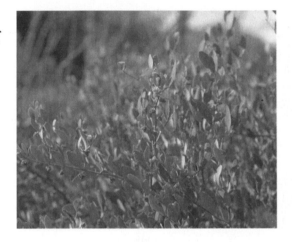

Figure 4.12 *Jojoba plant* (Simmondsia chinensis)

Uses of jojoba oil

- Good for moisturising the skin and hair
- Helps to relieve inflammation so is excellent for acne, eczema, psoriasis and arthritis.

Jojoba is an expensive oil so it is wise to use a small amount and mix it with another carrier oil such as sweet almond. It is generally safe to use.

Using the information on pages 114–17, research the oils and complete the table below.

Oil	Brief description	Uses	Additional Information
Sesame			
Mustard			
Olive			
Coconut			
Sweet almond			
Jojoba			

BRUSHING THE HAIR

Before carrying out a scalp oil massage or moisturising treatment you may wish to brush the client's hair, especially if hairspray is worn. There is a simple way to avoid discomfort to the client's scalp while brushing.

If the client has hair spray on the hair, this can be brushed out using a vent brush (Figure 4.13). Begin at the tips of the hair and brush until the roots are reached. If the hair is long, pick up a portion of hair, hold it firmly and allow about 2 inches to stick out from the bottom of your hand. Ensure this hand is always close to the client's head so the hair will not be tugged from the scalp at any time. Brush the hair and then release it from your hand and repeat again but this time with about four inches of hair sticking out from the hand. Continue to brush the hair in this manner until the roots are reached.

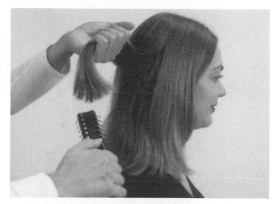

Figure 4.13   *How to brush long hair*

SCALP OIL MASSAGE

Choose an oil such as sweet almond and place it in a small bowl; it will pour more easily if it is warm. You may wish to put a towel around the client's shoulders and on their lap to prevent oil from staining clothes. Ensure that the bowl of oil is near you to avoid spillage on to the floor.

Traditionally the oils are applied to three different areas of the scalp.

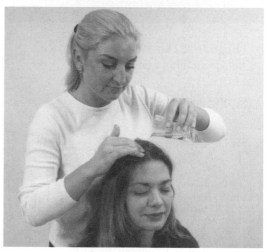

Figure 4.14a   *Applying oil to the hairline*

- The first area is just about an inch above the hairline at the front of the head. Ask the client to tip their head slightly back so that the oil does not get into the eyes. As it is poured, gently rub it into the scalp with circular movements using the fingertips of the other hand (Figure 14.4a).
- The oil is then applied to the crown of the head at the point where there is a circular pattern of hair growth. Gently pour the oil on to the crown. Using the fingertips of the other hand, massage it into the hair, following the direction of the hair-growth at the crown (Figure 14.4b).

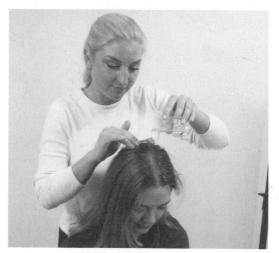

Figure 4.14b   *Applying oil to the crown of the head*

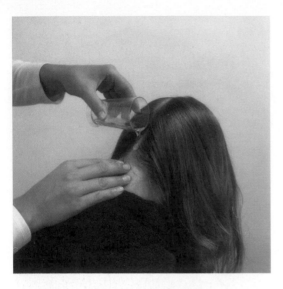

Figure 4.14c *Applying oil to the base of the occipital bone*

- Ask the client to tip their head forward. Apply the oil at the base of the occipital bone (Figure 14.4c). Using the fingertips of the other hand, create circular movements to spread the oil in this area. The scalp massage can now take place; ensure the oil is spread evenly over the scalp and hair.

The client should be advised to leave the oil on the hair for as long as possible, preferably about 10 hours.

Benefits of scalp oil massage

- Stimulates blood circulation, nourishing the scalp, which improves the condition of the scalp
- Loosens scalp muscles, relieving tension within them
- Conditions and moisturises dry hair and scalp.

Moisturising treatment for long hair or a particularly dry scalp

You will need:

- A bowl of oil such as sweet almond, preferably warm
- A hair brush and a tail comb
- A brush, preferably a tint brush as used in hairdressing but you can use another type
- Section clips, as used in hairdressing, but you can use hair clips or hair bands instead
- Plastic sheeting to put on the floor
- A protective gown, as used in hairdressing, but towels can be used instead
- A towel to wrap around the client's head
- A plastic cap to go on the head, such as is used during a perming treatment – or cling film can be used instead.

Both the floor and the client's clothing should be protected with plastic sheets, protective gown and towels. It may also be wise to ask the client to wear old clothing when coming for this treatment.

First, you may need to brush the client's hair so that it can easily be parted into sections. The client's hair needs to be divided into a 'hot cross bun' section (Figure 4.15). Use the section clips or hair bands to divide the hair into four sections. The clips will hold the sections in place.

Next, stand behind the client and begin working on one of the sections at the back of the head. Use the end of the tail comb and pick up a triangular portion of hair from that section near the top of the head. Place the brush in the oil, hold the portion of hair in one hand and with the other apply the oil to the hair in downward strokes. Give particular attention to the ends of the hair, especially if it is dry. Continue to work through the section of hair until it is all covered with oil, although not dripping. After you have finished the back two sections, move to the front of the client and work on the front two sections until all the hair is covered in oil.

You may want to offer this as an individual treatment to your client or include it in the Indian head massage treatment, although it may prove a little messy. If you are going to massage the head while the oil is on the hair it would be

Note

With the exception of the plastic sheet and cling film, all these products can be purchased at a hair and beauty wholesalers.

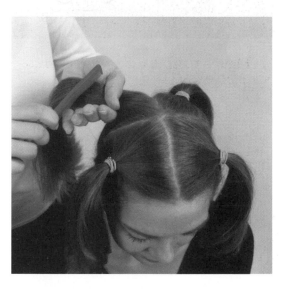

Figure 4.15 *Dividing hair into hot-cross-bun sections*

Note

There are different ways in which the oil can be applied to the hair. One way that is often used is to pour the oil through the hair while the client is lying on their back.

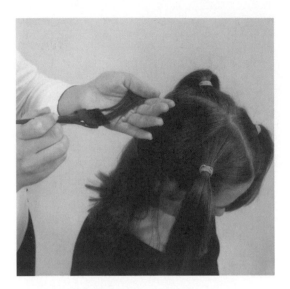

Figure 4.16 *Brushing oil on to the ends of long hair*

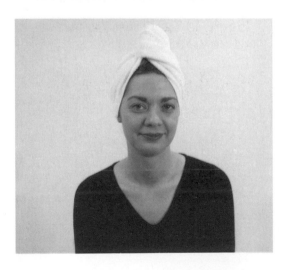

Figure 4.17 *Cover the client's head with a plastic cap and a towel*

advisable to carry out the back and arm massage first and then apply the oil. You can then proceed with the neck, scalp and facial massage (Chapter 5).

For an excellent moisturising treatment, place a plastic cap over the head to help keep in warmth and prevent any drips from the hair. Then wrap a towel around the head. The warmth will help to open the follicles so the oil can penetrate the hair more easily. Ensure that the client has a lift home as they may not want to walk to the car with a towel on their head! Ideally the client should leave the plastic cap on overnight and wash as normal in the morning. Hair grips can be used to secure the plastic cap overnight.

ESSENTIAL OILS

Traditionally in India, essential oils were not used during a head massage treatment but in the West the use of essential oils has become very popular, especially during massage treatments. The vegetable oils can be mixed with essential oils. Essential oils are extracted from leaves, petals, twigs, fruits and bark of plants. They can be purchased pre-blended from shops and wholesalers. Unless you are a qualified aromatherapist you should not blend the oils yourself.

It is best not to keep pre-blended oils for more than 6 months. Check them regularly to see if the oil looks cloudy and smell them to ensure that it has not gone off. The oils need to be kept in a dark, cool place away from sunlight.

A pure essential oil can enter the body within 20 minutes and stay in the bloodstream for over 24 hours. It enters the body through the hair follicles and the breath.

Table 4.1 overleaf will help you to choose essentials oils to suit your client's individual needs. If you are not a qualified aromatherapist you can buy pre-blended oils containing the essential oils stated in the table.

Note

Unless you are a qualified aroma-therapist you should not blend essential oils with carrier oils.

Self-test questions

Ask yourself the following self-test questions:

1. State five effects that massage has on the head, neck, face and shoulders.
2. What effect does an improved circulation to the scalp have on the skin and hair?
3. Name three benefits of scalp oil massage.
4. What considerations would you take into account while giving a scalp oil massage?
5. List four different oils used in Indian head massage and give a brief description of each.
6. Name four types of massage movements you have used while giving an Indian head massage.

Write down your answers on a sheet of paper. There are sample answers at the back of the book.

Table 4.1 Uses of essential oils

Essential oil	Uses	Special notes
Lemon	Headache High blood pressure Sore throat Thread veins Oily skin and hair	Phototoxic – client should avoid sunlight as skin will burn
Rosemary	Muscle stiffness Low blood pressure Poor circulation	Avoid using on people with high blood pressure or epilepsy
Ylang ylang	Slows down over-rapid breathing and heart rate Helps to reduce high blood pressure Dry and oily skin types Antidepressant and sedative	Using too high a concentration of ylang ylang can cause nausea and/or headache
Sandalwood	Greasy or dry hair, as balances production of sebum Useful for oily and acne skin types Helps treat dandruff Antidepressant and sedative	
Lavender	Dandruff Headache Nausea Aches and pains Acne Psoriasis Eczema/dermatitis Mature skin High blood pressure	
Chamomile	Aches and pains Acne Sensitive skin Psoriasis Eczema/dermatitis	
Black pepper	Aches and pains Poor circulation Toothache	Too much may overstimulate kidneys In high concentration may irritate skin

The Indian Head Massage Procedure

5

BEFORE YOU START

The therapist

It is important that the therapist presents a professional appearance and manner when carrying out an Indian head massage. Ideally a white tunic should be worn with white or dark trousers; ensure they are clean and ironed. Shoes must be clean and with a low heel. Long hair should be tied back and nails should be cut short. Jewellery should be kept to a minimum. If the therapist gives a bad first impression it is unlikely the client will come back.

It is important to adopt the correct posture when carrying out an Indian head massage. Always keep the back straight and the shoulders relaxed. When carrying out some of the massage movements on the back you may find you need to bend your knees rather than bending at the waist; this will help to prevent strain and injury to your back.

The client

Jewellery such as necklaces and earrings should be removed from the client prior to the massage. This will prevent the jewellery accidentally being broken and will help to ensure that the massage flows correctly.

If you are massaging the face, any make-up should be removed – perhaps you could ask the

Note

The whole Indian head massage treatment will take about 45 minutes, including the consultation.
Ensure that your client is aware of how long the treatment will take.

client to do this before coming. You can remove make-up with cleanser and some damp cotton wool pads; ensure the client is not allergic to the product.

How long will the treatment take?

An Indian head massage treatment will last for about 30 minutes. If a client has a condition such as an aching shoulder, which needs particular attention, you may find that you spend longer on that area than normal. If too much time is spent on one particular area (at the client's request) then you may have to shorten the massage on the face, otherwise you may run over time and be late for the next client.

The use of oils during treatment

The decision to use essential oils or other types of oil during the massage will be up to you and your client. If the client is going back to work after the appointment they may not want greasy-looking hair. Also, it is important to avoid getting oil on to the client's clothing during the treatment. Perhaps you can ask your client to wear non-valuable clothing, such as an old T-shirt. You can consider using towels to protect clothing. If your client prefers to remove their clothes you can provide a towel to wrap around them and work directly on the skin.

THE MASSAGE ROUTINE

Ensure your client is sitting in an upright position on a low-backed chair. The back of the chair should be no higher than the bottom of the client's shoulder blades (scapulae). Before the treatment starts, check that you have everything at hand, including a bolster or rolled up towel for when you are carrying out the face massage. If you

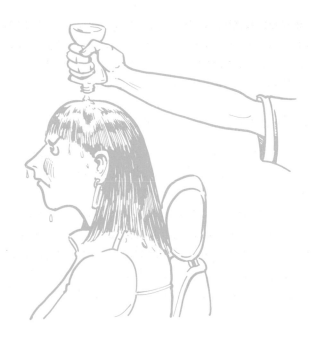

It is important to avoid covering the client in oil!

are using a trolley place any materials neatly on to it and make sure everything is clean.

- First carry out the consultation and ensure that your client signs the consultation form
- Make sure the client knows what to expect during treatment so they can relax
- Ensure the client is warm and comfortable; they may like to have a blanket on their legs or a pillow on their lap to rest their hands on
- Ensure that the client's feet are placed firmly on the floor, preferably with their shoes off
- Wash your hands; ideally the client should observe this
- Begin the massage by placing both hands on the client's shoulders
- Spend a few seconds mentally preparing yourself and try to breath at the same rate as your client.

Note

Try to maintain as much physical contact as you can throughout the treatment – do not lift your hands away from the body too often; instead, use stroking movements to link massage movements together.

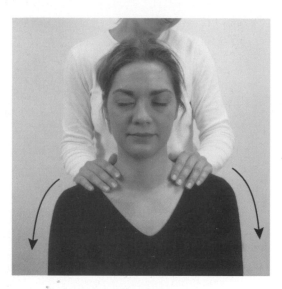

Figure 5.1 *Iron down*

Shoulders

1. Iron down

- Place both flat hands on the shoulders near the base of the client's neck.
- Mould your hands to the shape of the client's shoulders.
- Firmly glide hands along the top of the shoulders and down the upper arms.
- Gently stroke the hands back up the arms and return them back to the shoulders near the base of the neck.

(Repeat movement 2 times.)

2. Friction to shoulders

- Place both hands flat on the client's shoulders.
- Using the fingers of both hands gently rub each shoulder using quick, light side to side movements.
- Slide the hands to the upper part of the chest and gently rub using side to side movements.
- Slide the hands to the upper part of the back and repeat this movement.

(Repeat movement 3 times.)

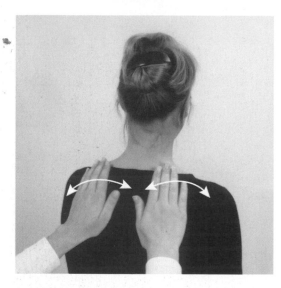

Figure 5.2 *Friction to shoulders*

Note

Friction to shoulders is gentle and soothing: it is good for releasing tension in the shoulders.

3. Thumb sweep around scapulae

- Place your thumbs at the base of the scapulae (shoulder blades).

- Using both thumbs sweep around the scapulae and across the shoulders (if you prefer you may use one thumb at a time and use the other hand to support the shoulder).

- At the shoulders lift the hands off and return the thumbs to the base of the scapulae.

(Repeat movement 4 times.)

4. Finger kneading around scapulae

- Stand to the left of the client.

- Place your left hand on the client's left shoulder (fingers pointing to the back of the client's body).

- Place the pads of the fingers of the right hand at the base of the right scapula.

- Create circular movements in a clockwise direction with the pads of the fingers. Work around the scapula up to the shoulders.

- Stroke your hand back to the base of scapula and repeat this movement 4 times.

- Swap sides and repeat movement with right hand on shoulder and use the fingers of left hand to create circular movements up and around the left scapula. Repeat this movement 4 times.

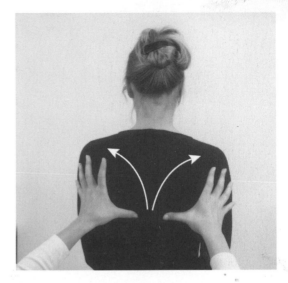

Figure 5.3   *Thumb sweep around scapulae*

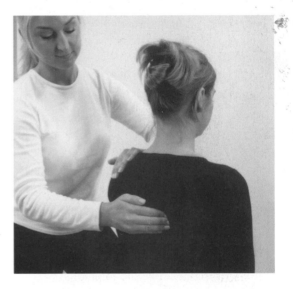

Figure 5.4   *Finger kneading around scapulae*

Note

Do not massage directly on to bony areas as it is uncomfortable for the client.

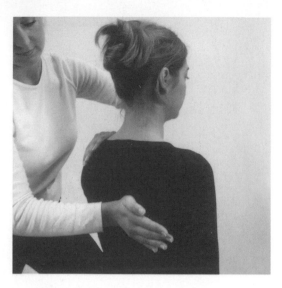

Figure 5.5 *Heel-of-hand knead around scapulae*

5. *Heel-of-hand knead around scapulae*

◊ Stand to the right side of the client with your right hand on the client's right shoulder, fingers of this hand pointing towards the back.

◊ Place the heel of the other hand at the base of the client's left scapula.

◊ Create small circular movements (fairly deep pressure) and work up and around the scapula, working on muscles only, not the bone.

◊ Lift hand off and return it to the base of the scapula and repeat 3 times.

◊ Swap sides and repeat this movement around the client's right scapula with the heel of your right hand.

Note

Deep pressure can be applied with the finger pads. Try to use the weight of your body effectively to help increase pressure, rather than using the muscles of the arms.

Note

Can you feel any knots or tension in the muscle being worked? Sometimes you may feel little granules, which indicate tension within the muscle; you will feel them dissolve as you massage.

6. Side-of-hands friction (sawing)

- Place the little finger sides of both hands anywhere on the upper back.

- Create a sawing action with hands, alternately moving each hand forwards and backwards.

- Work over the whole of the upper back and over the shoulders.

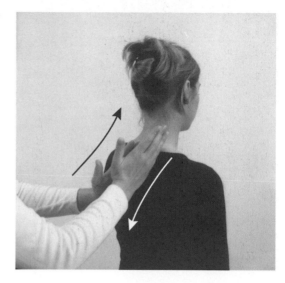

Figure 5.6 *Side-of-hands friction*

7. Hacking to upper back

- Place the little-finger sides of both hands at the top of the back, anywhere on the trapezius muscle.

- Fingers should not be completely straight but slightly cupped in shape.

- With loose wrists alternately chop with each hand, ensuring pressure is not too great (be gentle over bony areas).

- Work over the whole upper back and shoulder area.

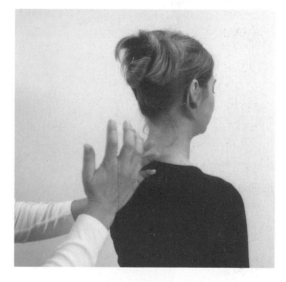

Figure 5.7 *Hacking to upper back*

Note

Practise this movement on a cushion.

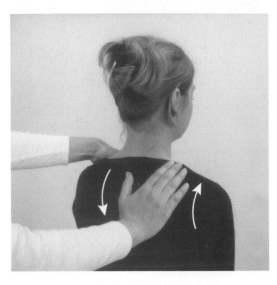

Figure 5.8 *Push and pull alternate shoulders*

8. Push and pull alternate shoulders

◊ Place both hands on client's shoulders.

◊ Slide right hand forwards so it is placed flat on the client's right upper chest region.

◊ Slide the left hand backwards so it is placed flat on the left side of the upper back.

◊ Gently push both hands at the same time so that the left shoulder moves forward and the right shoulder moves backwards so a gentle stretch is achieved. Repeat 3 times.

◊ Slide the right hand backwards so that it is placed on the client's back and the slide the left hand forward so that it is placed on the upper chest region. Push both hands at the same time and repeat the stretch. Repeat 3 times.

9. Shoulder pick-up and squeeze

◊ Place your hands on the client's shoulders, near the base of the neck, fingers pointing forwards and thumb facing the back of the body.

◊ Push the thumbs towards the fingers. Pick up and squeeze muscles of shoulders between your thumb and fingers and then release.

◊ Repeat this movement about four times working outwards from the neck and across the shoulders.

(Repeat whole sequence 3 times.)

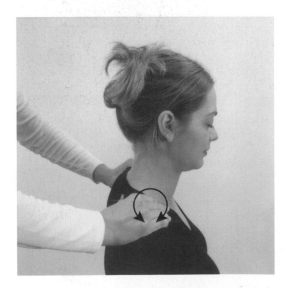

Figure 5.9 *Shoulder pick-up and squeeze*

10. Heel push to shoulders

- Cup hands over the client's shoulders, near the base of the neck.
- With the heel of the hands press then release. Use your body weight to create a deeper movement.
- Work from the base of the neck outwards across the shoulders and then stroke hands back again.

(Repeat the movement 3 times.)

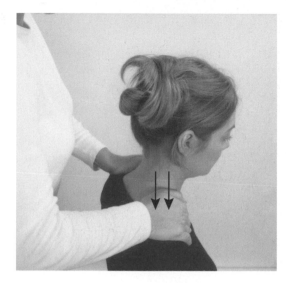

Figure 5.10 *Heel push to shoulders*

11. Circular heel-of-hand roll to shoulder

- Place both hands on the client's shoulders. The right hand should be near the base of the neck.
- Use the heel of the right hand to create circular movements to the top of the shoulder.
- Begin at the base of the neck and work outwards across the shoulders then back to the base of the neck.
- Repeat the movement with the left hand to the left shoulder.

(Repeat 3 times on each side.)

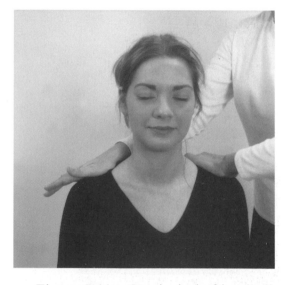

Figure 5.11 *Circular heel-of-hand roll to shoulder*

Note

If you can feel any knots, use a vibrations massage movement (your forearm muscles are contracted and small tremors are created with the pads of the first two fingers). This will help to disperse the knot (see page 110).

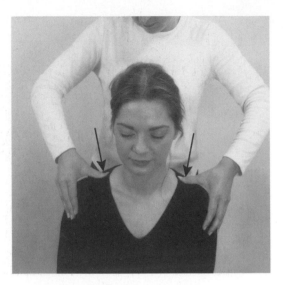

Figure 5.12 *Thumb push to shoulder*

12. Thumb push to shoulder

◊ Place the pads of your thumbs on the outer edge of the client's shoulders.

◊ Use the pads of your thumbs to push into the shoulder muscle. Release and move about 2 cm towards the base of the neck and again push, then release. Repeat this movement until you reach the neck area.

◊ Slide the thumbs to the outer edge of the shoulders but place them about 2 cm further back than last time, towards the back of the body. Push and release thumbs again until the neck area is reached.

◊ Repeat this movement until the whole of the top of the shoulders has been worked over.

13. Circular thumb knead to shoulders

◊ Place hands on each shoulder, near the base of the neck.

◊ Use the pads of the thumbs to create slow, circular, clockwise movements.

◊ Begin at the base of the neck and work outwards across the shoulders. Repeat this movement until the muscles of the upper back and shoulders have been massaged.

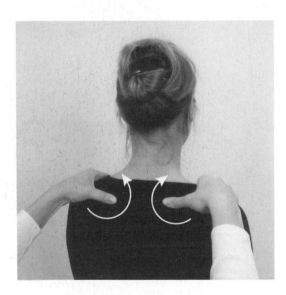

Figure 5.13 *Circular thumb knead to shoulders*

Note

Remember to keep your nails short!

Note

Try to work over the whole of the trapezius muscle. Can you feel any knots?

14. Iron down

- Place both hands on the client's shoulders, near the base of the neck.
- Firmly slide hands across the top of the shoulders and down the upper arms.
- Lift hands off at client's elbow and repeat the movement.

(Repeat the movement 3 times.)

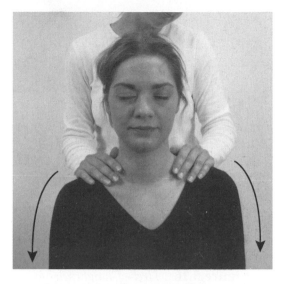

Figure 5.14   *Iron down*

Arm massage

15. Pick-up and squeeze to upper arms

- Place each hand at the top of one of the client's arms.
- Squeeze with the hand and then release.
- Slide the hands down the arms, alternately squeezing and releasing.
- When the elbow is reached, stroke back up the arms.

(Repeat the movement 2 times.)

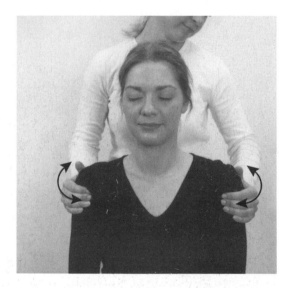

Figure 5.15   *Pick-up and squeeze to upper arms*

Note

Ask the client how the pressure feels – would they like lighter or deeper pressure?

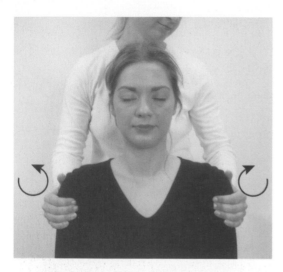

Figure 5.16 *Heel-of-hand circles to upper arms*

16. Heel-of-hand circles to upper arms

- Place your hands at the top of the client's arms, fingers pointing forwards.
- Use the heel of the hand to make circular movements.
- Work down the arms and back up again.
- Ensure that the whole of the upper arm (biceps and triceps) is massaged.

(Repeat movement 2 times.)

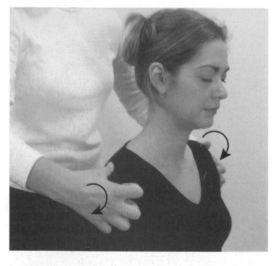

Figure 5.17 *Knuckling to upper arms*

17. Knuckling to upper arms

- Place your hands at the top of each arm.
- Make a loose fist with each hand, the fingers and knuckles slightly apart.
- Create circular movements with the fist, using the parts of the fingers about 2.5 cm down from the nail to massage and keeping the wrists loose.
- Work over the whole upper arm, particularly concentrating on the biceps and triceps.

Note

The upper arms can be quite sensitive so do not use too much pressure when massaging.

18. Forearm roll to tops of shoulders and upper arms

- Place the backs of the forearms on the client's shoulders near the base of the neck. Your palms should be facing upwards.

- Slowly slide the forearms across the shoulders, at the same time rolling the hands inwards so that the palms have turned to face downwards when they reach the tops of the arms.

- Stroke down each of the client's arms with the inside of the forearms.

(Repeat 3 times.)

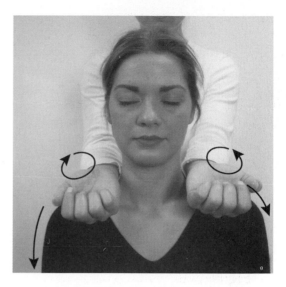

Figure 5.18 *Forearm roll to tops of shoulders and upper arms*

Neck

All the neck movements are carried out standing to the side of the client. You may wish to use oil for the neck massage.

19. Fingers-and-thumb slide

- Place one hand on the client's forehead to support the head.

- Place the fingers and thumb of the other hand on either side of the vertebrae, on the muscles of the neck.

- Slide the fingers and thumb up the neck to the occipital bone and then slide back down to the base of the neck. You do not need to swap sides for this movement.

(Repeat movement 4 times.)

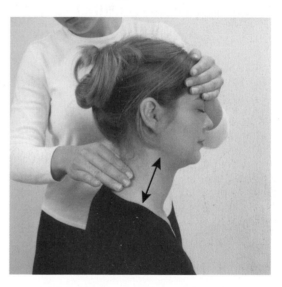

Figure 5.19 *Fingers-and-thumb slide*

Note

When massaging the neck ensure that you work to either side of the spine and not directly on it.

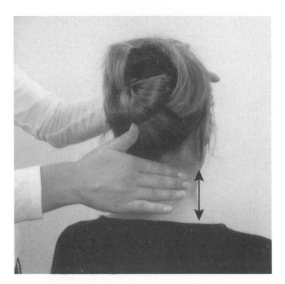

Figure 5.20 *Three-fingers rub to either side of neck*

20. Three-fingers rub to either side of neck

- Place one hand on the client's forehead to support the head.
- Use the first three fingers of the other hand and place them at the base of the client's neck.
- Gently rub the neck with the fingers creating small up-and-down movements.
- Work up and down one side of the neck and then work on the other side of the neck using the same hand.

(Repeat 2 times on each side of neck.)

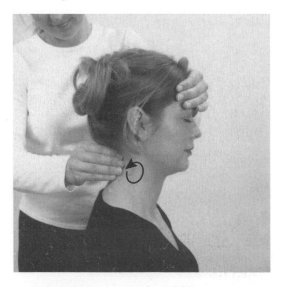

Figure 5.21 *Finger-and-thumb circles to either side of neck*

21. Finger-and-thumb circles to either side of neck

- Place one hand on the client's forehead to support the head.
- Place the thumb and fingers of the other hand at either side of the vertebrae at the base of the neck.
- The thumb and fingers slide gently forward to make a small, slow, circular movement and then return to the starting position. Repeat these finger-and-thumb circles and work slowly up to the occipital bone and back down the neck.

(Repeat this movement 4 times.)

Note

Be careful not to drag the skin if you are not using oil.

22. Finger-and-heel-of-hand grasp to neck

- Place one hand on the client's forehead to support the head.

- Use the heel of the other hand and fingers to cup and grasp the neck.

- Squeeze and release the muscles at the back of the neck.

- You do not need to swap sides for this movement.

(Repeat this movement 3 times.)

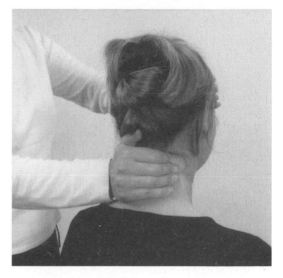

Figure 5.22 *Finger-and-heel-of-hand grasp to neck*

23. Heel-of-hand knead to neck

- Place one hand on the client's forehead to support the head.

- Place the heel of the other hand at the base of the neck to the right side of the spine.

- Apply gentle pressure to the neck, creating circular movements with the heel of the hand, and work up and down the right side of the neck for about 8 seconds.

- Repeat this movement to the left side of the neck using the same hand.

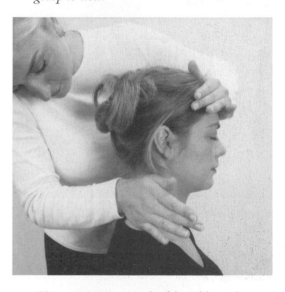

Figure 5.23 *Heel-of-hand knead to neck*

Note

If the neck is small, use your fingers and thumb to grasp the neck instead.

Note

If there is tension in the neck area, why not use vibration massage movements (see page 111)?

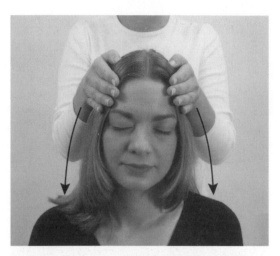

Figure 5.24 *Effleurage to head*

Head massage

24. Effleurage to head

- Stand behind the client.
- Place both hands on top of the client's head.
- Gently stroke hands alternately down the head.
- Repeat until the whole head has been worked.

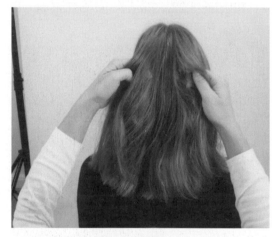

Figure 5.25 *Ruffling to hair*

25. Ruffling to hair

- Lightly place hands on top of head.
- Open the fingers and draw them through the hair.
- Create wave-like movements, working from the roots to the tips of the hair.

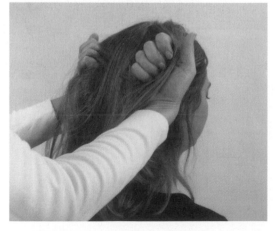

Figure 5.26 *Hair tugging*

26. Hair tugging

- Stand behind the client and place your hands on either side of their head.
- Turn hands over with palms facing upwards.
- Comb fingers into the hair.
- Close the fingers together locking the hair in between them.
- Gently tug at the hair and then release.
- Repeat until the whole head has been worked.

27. Friction to head

- Stand to the side of the client and support the forehead with one hand.

- Place the heel of the other hand at the base of the head (occipital bone).

- Make small, quick, side-to-side movements using the heel of the hand.

- Work from the base of the head up to the hairline at the forehead.

- Repeat until the whole head has been worked.

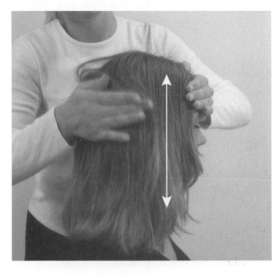

Figure 5.27   *Friction to the head*

28. Three-finger rub to head

- Stand to the side of the client and support the forehead with one hand.

- Place the other hand on the occipital bone.

- Using the first three fingers briskly rub the head, making side-to-side movements.

- Work from the base of the head up to the hairline at the forehead.

- Repeat until the whole head has been worked.

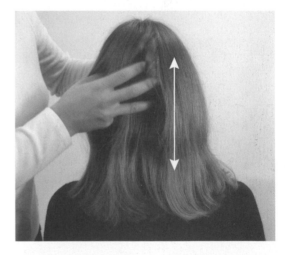

Figure 5.28   *Three-finger rub to the head*

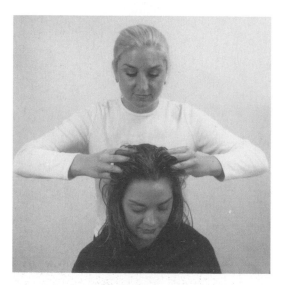

Figure 5.29 *Shampooing to head*

29. Shampooing

- Place your hands on either side of the scalp.
- Spread out the fingers and with the pads of the fingers make small, brisk, circular movements as if applying shampoo to the hair and scalp.
- Ensure that the whole scalp is worked.

30. Pétrissage to the scalp

- Place your hands on either side of the scalp.
- Spread out the fingers and with the pads of the fingers glued to the scalp make small, circular movements.
- Lift the fingers away and move to another part of the scalp and work that area, ensuring the whole of the scalp is massaged.
- Complete the head massage by ruffling the hair.

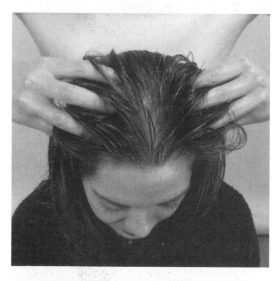

Figure 5.30 *Pétrissage to scalp*

Note

This is an excellent movement for releasing tension in the scalp muscles.

Facial

Place a bolster or rolled up towel behind your client's neck to help support it. You will still be standing behind the client to carry out the facial massage.

Note

This movement is good for relieving headaches and tension.

31. Effleurage to forehead

- Stand behind the client and use your body to keep the towel in position behind the neck.
- Use alternate palms to stroke slowly up the forehead.
- Work from the right side of the forehead to the left and then to the centre, ensuring that the whole area is worked.

(Repeat this movement 16 times.)

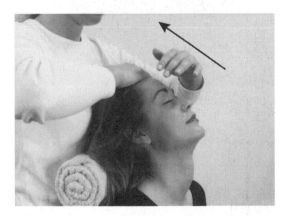

Figure 5.31 *Effleurage to forehead*

32. Pressure points to forehead

- Place the middle finger of one hand about 1 cm up from the bridge of the nose.
- Place the middle finger of the other hand on top of that finger to reinforce the movement (no. 1).
- Press and release the fingers and then slide about 1 cm upwards and repeat movement (no. 2).
- Repeat this movement up the forehead until the hairline is reached (no. 3).
- Place middle fingers 2 cm from the top centre of the forehead on either side (no. 4) Press and release fingers.
- Move middle fingers about 1 cm downwards (no. 5) Press and release.
- Slide the fingers down to the final pressure point (no. 6), which is just above each eyebrow.

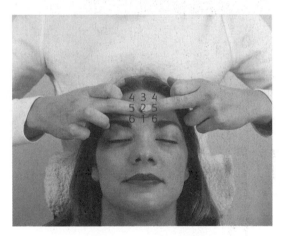

Figure 5.32 *Pressure points to forehead*

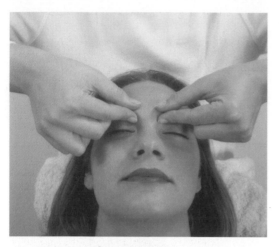

Figure 5.33 *Eyebrow squeeze*

33. Eyebrow squeeze

- Begin at the part of the eyebrow nearest to the centre of the face.
- Use the first finger and thumb of each hand and gently pinch the tissues of the eyebrow.
- Work slowly across the eyebrows continually squeezing and releasing.

(Repeat whole movement 3 times.)

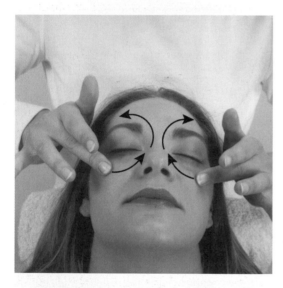

Figure 5.34 *Eye circles with middle finger*

34. Eye circles with middle finger

- Place your middle fingers at the outer corners of the client's eyes.
- Gently slide fingers under the eyes and up around the bridge of the nose.
- Bring fingers up and over eyebrows, creating full circles around each eye.

(Repeat 3 times.)

Note

This is a good movement to help unblock the sinuses.

35. Pressure to cheekbones

- Place your middle fingers on each side of the client's nose.
- Following the crescent shape of the cheekbones press and release with the middle fingers. Work the top of the cheekbones until you reach the temples. Slide the fingers back to each side of the nose.
- Repeat this movement a little lower down on the cheekbones and then finally work along the lower edge of the cheekbones.

(Repeat whole movement once only.)

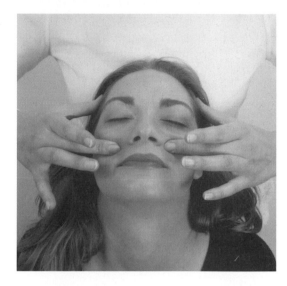

Figure 5.35 *Pressure to cheekbones*

36. Finger-and-thumb squeeze along jawbone

- Place your thumbs on the client's chin and your index fingers beneath the chin.
- Apply pressure and release.
- Slide fingers about 1 cm outwards and repeat pressures.
- Work from the chin to the top of the jaw bone.

(Repeat this movement 3 times.)

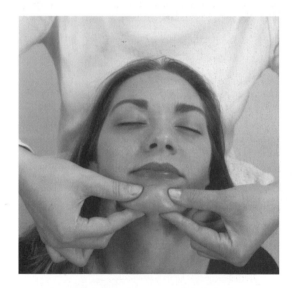

Figure 5.36 *Finger-and-thumb squeeze along jawbone*

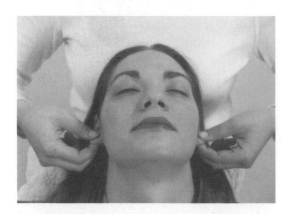

Figure 5.37 *Circular finger kneading to ear*

37. Circular finger kneading to ear

◊ Press your thumbs on the front of the client's ear lobes and the index fingers on the back of the lobes, your right hand working on the client's right ear and the left hand working on the left ear.

◊ Make small, circular movements with the thumb and finger. As you work up the ears you may have to swap over the finger and thumb and use the finger on the front of the ear and the thumb on the back to massage.

◊ Work up to the top of the ears and back down again.

(Repeat movement 3 times.)

38. Circular finger kneading to jaw bone

◊ Place your fingers on either side of the client's face where the jaw bones meet.

◊ Use the pads of the first three fingers to make slow, small, circular movements.

(Repeat movement for about 10 seconds.)

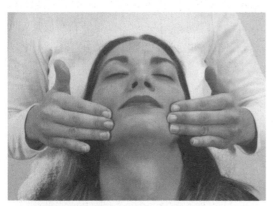

Figure 5.38 *Circular finger kneading to jaw bone*

Note

Even though their eyes are closed many clients report seeing vibrant colours such as purple and orange while the chakras are worked. For information on chakras see Chapter 7.

39. Chakra balancing

● Interlock the fingers of your hands. Place the hands about 3 cm from the client's throat – do not place hands directly on the throat (Figure 5.39a).

● Holds the hands in this position for about 10 seconds.

● Move the hands, still interlocked, up to the client's forehead and hold for about 10 seconds (Figure 5.39b).

● Move the interlocked hands up to the crown of the head, so that the palms are now facing downwards. Hold for about 10 seconds (Figure 5.39c).

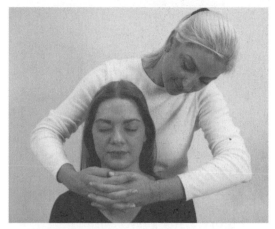

Figure 5.39a   *Chakra balancing – throat*

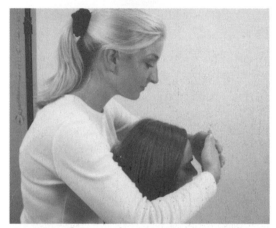

Figure 5.39b   *Chakra balancing – forehead*

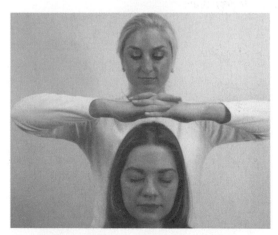

Figure 5.39c   *Chakra balancing – crown*

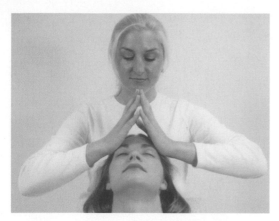

Figure 5.40 *Prayer effleurage*

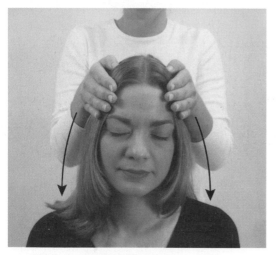

Figure 5.41 *Effleurage to head*

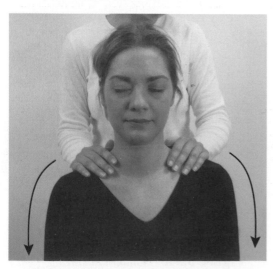

Figure 5.42 *Iron down*

40. Prayer effleurage

◊ Form your hands into a prayer position and then place them on the client's forehead so that the bases of your palms are touching the centre of the client's forehead.

◊ With the hands still in a prayer position, gently slide hands apart and downwards, so that each hand strokes either side of the forehead. Slide the hands back up again and return them to the prayer position. Repeat this movement 3 times

◊ With hands still in the prayer position place the base of the palms on the client's chin.

◊ Slide the hands apart and outwards until they reach the ears. Repeat this movement 3 times.

41. Effleurage to head

◊ Place both hands on the top of the client's head.

◊ Gently stroke the head with the hands, working downwards to tidy the hair.

(Repeat 2 times.)

42. Iron down

◊ Place both hands flat on the client's shoulders near the base of the neck.

◊ Mould your hands to the shape of the client's shoulders.

◊ Firmly glide hands along the top of the shoulders and down the upper arms.

◊ Gently stroke the hands back up the arms and return the hands back to the shoulders near the base of the neck.

(Repeat 2 times.)

Leave your hands on the client's shoulders for a few seconds. Slowly leave the client and observe them and ask them how they feel. Perhaps you could ask if they would like a drink of water. After the client has drunk the water you can give aftercare advice and then book their next appointment. (See Chapter 6 for aftercare advice).

(See Chapter 6 for aftercare advice).

Task 5.1

To fill in the table below, you will need to study the Indian head massage routine and decide whether the massage movements used during the treatment is a form of effleurage, pétrissage or tapotement.

Indian head massage element	Type of massage movement
Iron down	Effleurage
Finger kneading around scapulae	
Heel-of-hand knead around scapulae	
Hacking to upper back	
Shoulder pick-up and squeeze	
Thumb push to shoulders	
Circular thumb knead to shoulders	
Pick-up and squeeze to upper arms	
Heel-of-hand circles to upper arms	
Knuckling to upper arms	
Fingers-and-thumb slide	
Finger-and-heel-of-hand grasp to neck	
Eye circles with middle finger	
Finger-and-thumb squeeze along jawbone	
Circular finger kneading to jaw bone	

Ask yourself the following self-test questions:

1. What two questions might you ask your client to answer to determine whether the treatment was successful?
2. What non-verbal feedback might indicate that a client was happy with the treatment?
3. Why is feedback from the client important to the therapist?
4. Name two ways in which you can judge whether the treatment was effective.
5. How long does it take to carry out a full Indian head massage treatment?
6. Why does the Indian head massage need to be carried out in a set time?
7. Name three precautions you must take to avoid cross-infection while giving an Indian head massage.

Write down your answers on a sheet of paper. There are sample answers at the back of the book.

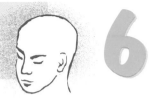

AFTERCARE ADVICE

Aftercare advice should be given directly after the treatment. It is important for the client to follow aftercare advice so that the full benefit of the treatment can be gained.

- The client should be encouraged to rest and relax after the treatment. This ensures that the body is able to heal itself sufficiently.

- The client should drink plenty of water (mineral or tap) or herbal tea to help speed up the removal of toxins from the body.

- Coffee, tea and cola should be avoided as they contain caffeine. Caffeine is a stimulant and therefore will not help the client to relax.

- The client should not smoke or drink alcohol for about 24 hours as the treatment is a detoxifying one and smoking and drinking will reintroduce toxins into the body.

- Heavy meals should be avoided after treatment as blood is diverted to the gut to help with the digestion of the food. The demands of digestion will divert energy away from the healing processes. Light meals such as fruit and vegetables will make an ideal snack.

- It may be wise to ask clients to wait for about 10 minutes after the treatment before driving home, especially if they feel sleepy.

7

THE CHAKRA SYSTEM

The Indian head massage routine includes chakra balancing work. The body has seven major chakras: ⑦ crown, ⑥ brow (third eye), ⑤ throat, ④ heart, ③ solar plexus, ② hara (sacrum) and ① base (root). An important part of Indian head massage is working with the higher chakras, the crown (*sahasrara*), third eye (*ajna*) and throat (*vishuddha*). Minor chakras are also found in the feet, on the palms of the hands and at joints.

The chakras are centres of energy that are located about an inch away from the body and should ideally spin in a clockwise direction. Each chakra resembles a flower and its petals represent energy channels through which energy passes. Each chakra has a different number of petals. The energy (*prana*) for the chakras is supplied from the universe. *Prana* is an Indian word meaning 'life-force energy'. It enters the body through these energy centres. To ensure health, all the chakras need to be open, unblocked and in balance with each other.

HIGHER CHAKRAS

The crown chakra is called the master chakra and can help to open up and balance the six other chakras of the body. It is important that this chakra is not blocked, otherwise energy will not be able to run freely from all the other chakras to it.

Working with this chakra will cause energy to be sent to where it is needed in the body and so promote healing. The crown chakra is the place through which the universe sends its energy into the body.

Note

Chakra is an ancient Indian word meaning 'wheel of light'.

Note

Some people can see chakras and describe them as spinning whirlpools of energy.

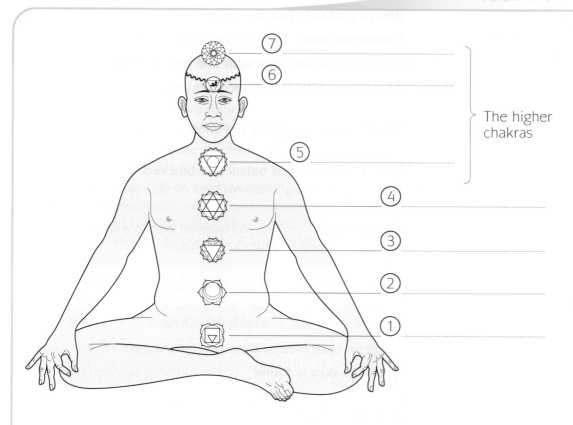

Figure 7.1   *The Chakras*

Label the diagram in Figure 7.1, matching the numbers to the numbered terms in the text opposite.

Remember that only qualified aromatherapists should blend essential oils. Unqualified aromatherapists will need to buy preblended oils from shops or wholesalers.

The solar plexus – third chakra

Where chakra is found – 5 cm above the navel

Concerned with – personality, feelings and emotional strength

Colour it is associated with and responds to – yellow

Endocrine gland it is associated with – the pancreas

Effects when balanced and unblocked – the person will be confident and responsible, with feelings of peace and inner harmony, and have high self-esteem

Effects when out of balance or blocked – the person will have a low sense of self-worth and be gloomy, bad-tempered, hyperactive and stubborn

Essential oils – Lavender oil has a calming, relaxing and balancing effect on hyperactive third chakras. It also helps to dissolve negative bottled-up emotions. Rosemary is useful for balancing the solar plexus chakra. Juniper strengthens will-power and increases self-worth. It helps to restore confidence and ease the fear of failure.

The hara (sacral chakra) – second chakra

Where chakra is found – 5 cm below the navel

Concerned with – relationships, especially with the opposite sex

Colour it is associated with and responds to – orange

Endocrine gland it is associated with – reproductive organs (females: ovaries, males: testes)

Effects when balanced and unblocked – the person will exhibit a zest for life and will feel sexual and attractive

Effects when out of balance or blocked – the person will suffer from sexual problems, lack of self-love and mood swings

Essential oils – ylang ylang is a well known aphrodisiac. Its smell makes you feel safe and helps to dissolve pent-up emotions and anger. In the Far East, sandalwood oil is often used to increase sexual energy.

Base or root chakra – first chakra

Where chakra is found – at the base of the spine

Concerned with – connection to mother earth, health and survival

Colour it is associated with and responds to – red

Endocrine gland it is associated with – the adrenal glands

Effects when balanced and unblocked – the person will show good health, optimism and enthusiasm for life and will feel safe and secure

Effects when out of balance or blocked – fearful, disorganised and possessive

Essential oils – palmarosa encourages feelings of security. Patchouli helps to unblock this chakra.

Note

Did you notice that the colours of the chakras are the same as the colours of the rainbow?

UNBALANCED CHAKRAS

Any type of negative stress can cause a chakra to become blocked or thrown out of balance. It can occur because of upset, shock or fear. An imbalance in one energy centre can affect the others, especially those closest to it; for example, if you suffer an upsetting experience the heart chakra is affected, which may cause you to have a bad stomach (solar plexus chakra) and you may find it difficult to talk (throat chakra).

When the chakras lose their ability to work harmoniously with each other they become unbalanced. Imbalances or blockages can be eased or corrected by contact with an energy that nourishes, or vibrates at a frequency beneficial to the chakra. To help rebalance these chakras the hands can be placed over the three higher chakras to help the energy to flow freely. Balancing means helping a chakra to achieve proper functioning so that it is not too open or closed. When in a balanced state, a person can remain calm and centred in any situation. When out of balance, people tend to withdraw, or be overwhelmed, or lose control of their emotions.

Reporting of Injuries, Diseases and Dangerous Occurrences Regulations (RIDDOR) 1995

Minor accidents should be entered into a record book, stating what occurred and what action was taken. Ideally all concerned should sign. If as a result of an accident at work anyone is off work for more than 3 days, or someone is seriously injured, has a type of occupational disease certified by the doctor, or even dies, a report should be sent to the local authority Environmental Health Department as soon as possible.

The Employer's Liability Act 1969

Employers must take out insurance policies in case of claims by employees for injury, disease or illness related to the workplace.

A certificate must be displayed at work to show that the employer has this insurance.

The Local Government Act 1982

Bylaws are laws made by your local council. Workplace bylaws are primarily concerned with hygiene and different councils around the country have different ones. You will probably find that there is no bylaw in your area relating to Indian head massage. However, advice can be sought from your local Environmental Health Officer.

Industry codes of practice for hygiene in salons and clinics

The Vocational Training Charitable Trust, in association with the Federation of Holistic Therapists, publishes a code of practice. This is concerned with hygiene in the salon and gives guidelines for the therapist. Local bylaws also contain these guidelines to ensure good hygienic practice and avoid cross-infection.

Performing Rights

Some therapists like to play relaxing music while giving a treatment. Any music played in waiting or treatment rooms is considered to be a public performance. If you play music you may need to purchase a licence from Phonographic Performance Ltd (PPL) or the Performing Rights Society (PRS). These organisations collect the performance fees and give the money to performers and record companies. If you do not buy a licence, legal action may be taken against you.

However, many composers are not members of the PPL or PRS and so no fee need be paid. Also, if the composer has been dead for 70 years, the music is no longer copyright and only the performer will need to be paid. To find out if you will need a licence to play a particular piece of music, contact the supplier.

The Data Protection Act 1998

Any information about an individual such as a client that is stored on a computer must be registered with the Data Protection Register. The Data Protection Act requires this information to be used by the therapist only and not given to anyone else without the client's permission. This act does not apply to manual records, such as record cards stored in boxes.

The Consumer Protection Act 1987

This Act provides the customer with protection when they purchase goods or services. Products must be safe for use on the client during the treatment, or to be sold as a retail product.

Before the Consumer Protection Act was passed, if a person was injured by using a product they had to prove that the manufacturer had been negligent in some way in

Task 2.10

	Brief description	Is it infectious?
Ringworm (*Tinea corporosis*)	Red, scaly, circular patches which spread outwards. Centre of patch heals forming a ring shape. Sometimes caught through touching animals.	Yes
Scalp ringworm (*Tinea capilis*)	Infects the epidermis, forming grey, scaly areas. Sometimes breakage of hairs.	Yes
Ringworm of the beard (*Tinea barbae*)	Scaly patches with partial hair loss.	Yes

Task 2.11

	Brief description	Is it infectious?
Scabies	Wavy greyish lines can be seen commonly in webs of the fingers and crease of the elbow. It is very itchy.	Yes
Hair lice	Parasite lives in hair and lays eggs. Eggs attach to the hair close to the scalp. Very itchy.	Yes

	Brief description	Is it infectious?
Chloasma	**Areas of increased pigmentation, often seen on the face. May be due to sunburn, pregnancy or contraceptive pill.**	**No**
Vitiligo	**Complete loss of colour in areas of the skin. Cause is unknown. Affected areas are very sensitive to sunlight and burn easily.**	**No**
Albinism	**Skin, hair and eyes lack colour.**	**No**
Freckles (ephelides)	**Small, pigmented areas of skin. UV rays from sunlight stimulate the production of melanin and darker freckles, or create new ones.**	**No**
Lentigo	**Slightly raised, brown, pigmented areas of skin, which do not darken when exposed to UV light. Common on face and hands.**	**No**
Naevus	**Purplish-pink birthmark, often found on face and neck. Can vary in size.**	**No**
Port wine stain	**Large areas of dilated capillaries, reddish in colour, mostly occurring on head and neck.**	**No**

	Brief description	Is it infectious?
Psoriasis	Skin cells reproduce too quickly causing thickened patches of skin that are red, dry and itchy and covered in silvery scales. Can affect any part of the body. Cause is unknown although hereditary factors and stress play a part.	No
Skin tags	Loose, fibrous tissue that protrudes out from the skin and is mainly brown in colour.	No
Basal and squamous cell carcinomas	Account for 95% of all skin cancers. Usually found on areas of the body exposed to the sun. Begin as small, shiny, rounded lumps and form into ulcers. Brought on by U.V. light and are usually found in fair skinned people.	No
Melanoma	A skin growth due to over activity of the melanocytes caused by excessive exposure to the sun. Often occur at site of a mole. Although rare it is extremely dangerous. It is irregular in outline, patchy in colour, itchy or sore and may bleed.	No

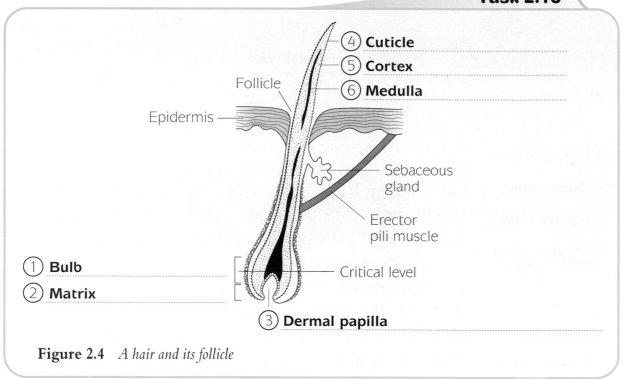

Figure 2.4   *A hair and its follicle*

Task 2.17

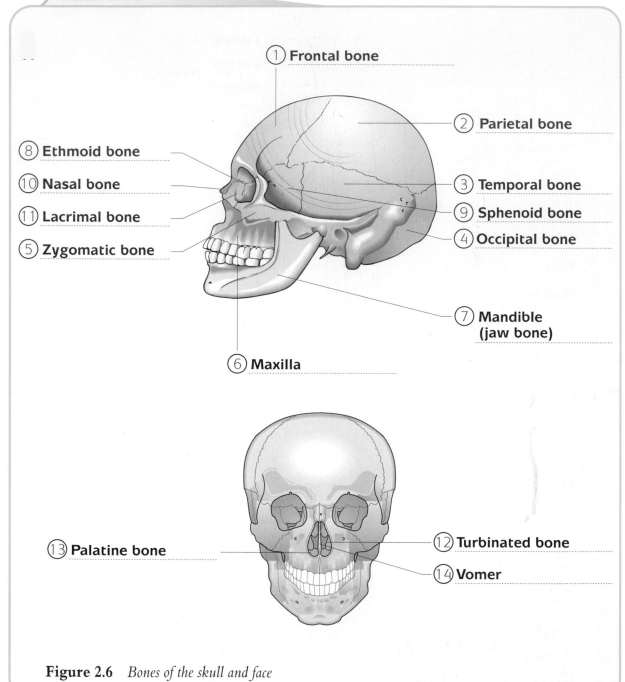

① **Frontal bone**

② **Parietal bone**

⑧ **Ethmoid bone**

⑩ **Nasal bone**

⑪ **Lacrimal bone**

⑤ **Zygomatic bone**

③ **Temporal bone**

⑨ **Sphenoid bone**

④ **Occipital bone**

⑦ **Mandible (jaw bone)**

⑥ **Maxilla**

⑬ **Palatine bone**

⑫ **Turbinated bone**

⑭ **Vomer**

Figure 2.6 *Bones of the skull and face*

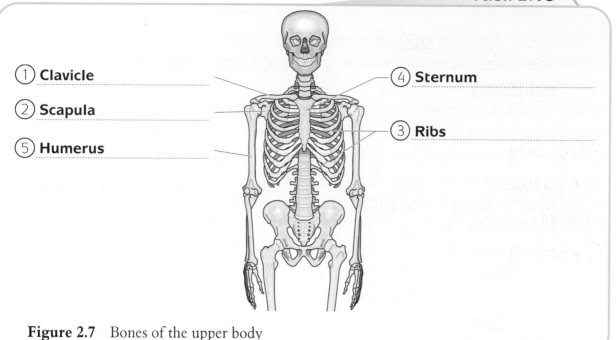

① **Clavicle**

② **Scapula**

⑤ **Humerus**

④ **Sternum**

③ **Ribs**

Figure 2.7   Bones of the upper body

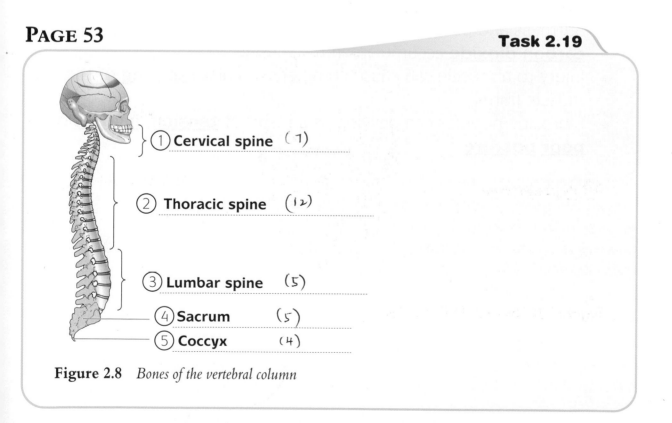

① **Cervical spine** (7)

② **Thoracic spine** (12)

③ **Lumbar spine** (5)

④ **Sacrum** (5)

⑤ **Coccyx** (4)

Figure 2.8   *Bones of the vertebral column*

- There are over **600** muscles in the body.
- The three types of muscle are **involuntary**, **cardiac** and **voluntary**.
- Skeletal muscles are an example of **voluntary** muscles.
- When a muscle contracts the thinner filaments, **actin**, slide in between the thicker filaments, called **myosin**.
- A **motor** nerve stimulates the muscle to contract.
- Muscle **tone** is the slight tension in which the muscles are continually held.
- When there is a low degree of muscle tone, the muscles are said to be **flaccid**.
- When there is a high degree of muscle tone, the muscles are said to be **spastic**.
- Muscle fatigue occurs when there is insufficient **oxygen** and **glucose**.
- Stiffness and pain results when the waste products **lactic acid** and **carbon dioxide** accumulate in the muscle.
- Injury to a muscle can cause complete or partial **tearing** of the muscle fibres.
- Fibrositic nodules can develop as a result of **tension**, **injuries** or **poor posture**.

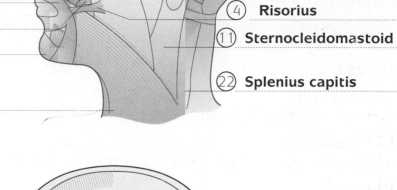

① Frontalis

② Corrugator
⑥ Orbicularis oculi

⑨ Orbicularis oris
③ Buccinator
⑧ Mentalis

⑫ Platysma

⑩ Temporalis
⑲ Occipitalis
⑦ Zygomaticus major
⑤ Masseter
④ Risorius
⑪ Sternocleidomastoid

㉒ Splenius capitis

⑭ Levator labii superioris

⑮ Depressor anguli oris

⑱ Procerus
⑰ Nasalis
⑬ Levator anguli oris
⑳ Pterygoid
㉑ Triangularis
⑯ Depressor labii inferioris

Figure 2.12 *Muscles of the face and neck*

Back of body

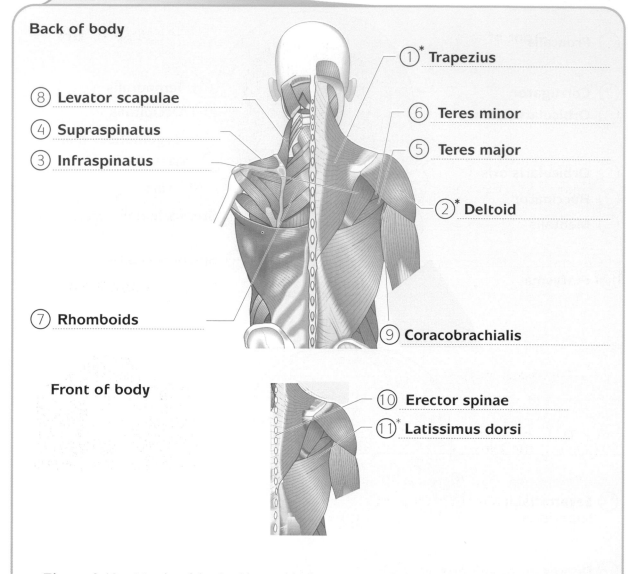

① * **Trapezius**

⑧ **Levator scapulae**

⑥ **Teres minor**

④ **Supraspinatus**

⑤ **Teres major**

③ **Infraspinatus**

② * **Deltoid**

⑦ **Rhomboids**

⑨ **Coracobrachialis**

Front of body

⑩ **Erector spinae**

⑪ * **Latissimus dorsi**

Figure 2.13 *Muscles of the shoulders and back.*
⋆ These are the muscles you will be working directly over when massaging.
The other muscles are deeper.

Task 2.23

Front of arm   Back of arm

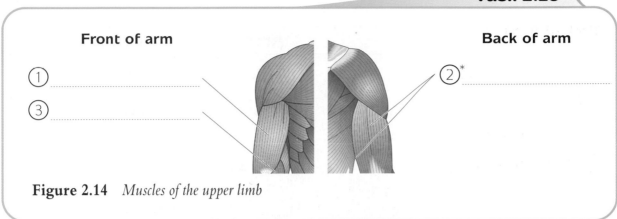

① ....

③ ....

②* ....

Figure 2.14 *Muscles of the upper limb*

Task 2.24

① **Pectoralis major** ....

② **Serratus anterior** ....

Figure 2.15   Muscles of the chest

	Arteries	Veins
Thickness of walls	**Thick**	**Thin**
Pressure of blood	**High**	**Low**
Do they have valves?	**No**	**Yes**
Blood carried oxygenated/ deoxygenated?	**Oxygenated**	**Deoxygenated**
Blood to heart/away from heart?	**Away from heart**	**To heart**
How blood is moved along vessels	**Pumping action of the heart**	**Relies on movement of the body**
Deep-seated or near surface of body?	**Deep seated**	**Nearer surface of the body**

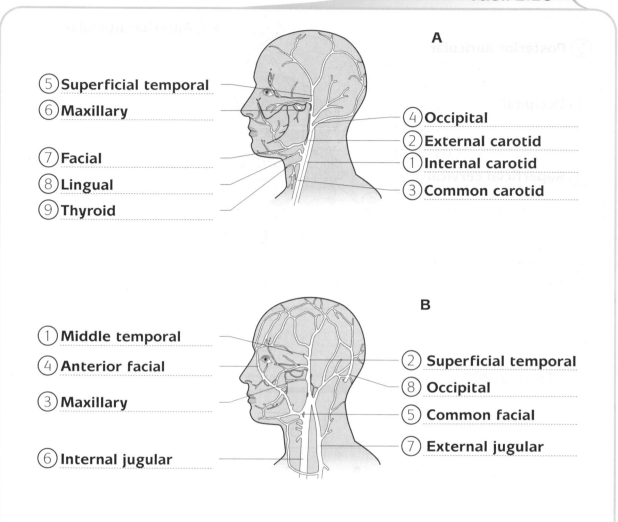

⑤ Superficial temporal
⑥ Maxillary

⑦ Facial
⑧ Lingual
⑨ Thyroid

A

④ Occipital
② External carotid
① Internal carotid
③ Common carotid

B

① Middle temporal
④ Anterior facial
③ Maxillary
⑥ Internal jugular

② Superficial temporal
⑧ Occipital
⑤ Common facial
⑦ External jugular

Figure 2.22 *Blood vessels of the head and neck:* **A** *arteries;* **B** *veins*

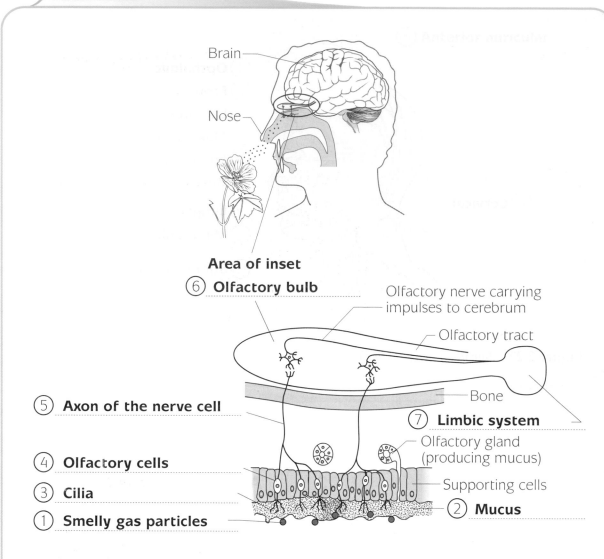

Figure 2.28 *The olfactory system*

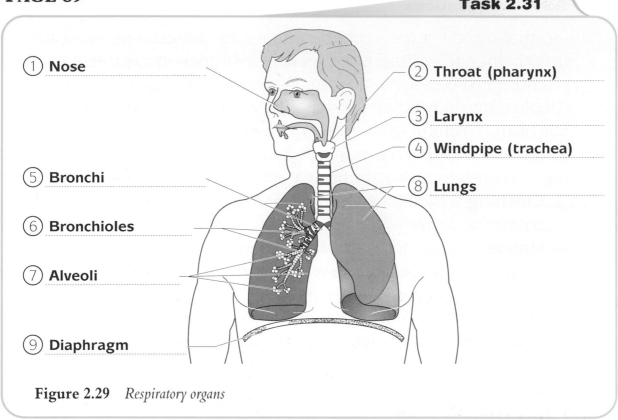

① **Nose**

② **Throat (pharynx)**

③ **Larynx**

④ **Windpipe (trachea)**

⑤ **Bronchi**

⑧ **Lungs**

⑥ **Bronchioles**

⑦ **Alveoli**

⑨ **Diaphragm**

Figure 2.29 *Respiratory organs*

PAGE 101

List all the contraindications to Indian head massage:

Any recent head or neck injury	**Thrombosis or embolism**
Migraine	**Diabetes**
Epilepsy	**Spastic conditions**
Recent haemorrhage	**Dysfunction of the nervous**
High blood pressure	**system**
Low blood pressure	**Skin disorders/scalp infections**
Severe bruising, cuts or abrasions in treatment area	**Recent operations**

Self-test questions

1. So that the client feels confident that they will get a professional treatment and will therefore return for further appointments.

2. To appear professional the therapist should be clean and smart. Unpleasant body odours and a dirty treatment room will deter the client from returning for further treatments. (Subconsciously, a client will think 'How can this therapist look after me if she cannot be bothered to look after herself and her treatment room?')

3. **Clothing** – should be clean and ironed. Ideally, a white tunic top should be worn.

   Hands – hands and nails should be clean. Nails should be short. No varnish (unless clear) should be worn. Cover any cuts, warts, etc. with a plaster.

   Hair – should be clean, with long hair tied back.

   Jewellery – a minimum amount of jewellery should be worn – only a wedding ring and, ideally, one pair of studs in the ears.

   Shoes – flat shoes (not trainers) should be worn. Ensure that they are clean and comfortable to wear.

4. Greeting the client with a smile will ensure that they feel welcome, and being polite to them will ensure that you appear professional and friendly.

5. Gives a professional appearance
   Helps protect your clothing from oil spillage.

6. The record card should be clearly written in case you need to contact the client or perhaps another therapist needs to read the card if they are also treating that particular client. The information needs to be accurate in case a client has a contraindication to the treatment, in which case it would be unwise to carry out the massage.

7. If the staff feel unsafe at work they will not feel happy and so will probably not give a good Indian head massage treatment. If the client feels unsafe they will not relax during the treatment and will probably not come back again.

8. ◦ **The services you offer –** so that you do not mislead the client and they know exactly what treatments you provide.

◦ **Price –** clients should be aware of the price of treatment prior to it being carried out so they know exactly how much to pay. They may be irritated if they feel that they have been misled about cost.

◦ **The Length of time taken for treatment –** the client may have other appointments to attend or may feel cheated if the time taken is shorter than they anticipated.

◦ **Products sold –** clients need to know how to use products, so that they are effective and safe. They must be clear about the purpose of a product that is sold to them and must not be misled in any way.

9. By establishing the reasons for a client coming for treatment, you can treat that client effectively to ensure that the Indian head massage will meet their expectations. They will thus be more likely to return for further treatments.

10. Explain that it is a safe treatment and that they will gain many health benefits. Ensure that the client knows what the treatment entails.

11. **Treatment plan**

Client name: Date of treatment:
Madeline Edwards   16 December

What are the client's expectations of treatment?

◦ To be relaxed
◦ To reduce tension in her shoulders
◦ To have a good night's sleep.

What are the treatment objectives?

◦ To spend extra time on shoulders to treat tension within the muscles
◦ To help relieve tension in her shoulders, neck and head areas, which may help prevent her from getting tension headaches

◆ To help the client to relax so that she can feel less stressed and have a restful night's sleep.

What oils are used, if any?

Sweet almond oil. Pre-blended aromatherapy oils containing lavender and chamomile to help relieve tension in the muscles, aid relaxation and help calm her so that she will sleep well tonight.

Any special needs?

Discuss relaxation techniques with the client, which will hopefully help prevent the tension headaches.

12. The client's body language will inform you of many emotions, such as nervousness, unhappiness or perhaps anger, so by reacting positively to it you will be able to deal with the client more effectively and they will leave the therapy room feeling satisfied and therefore return for further massages.

13. If the client has a local contraindication such as a bruise, cut or cold sore, it can be worked round. If a client has a general contraindication, such as high blood pressure, their doctor's advice should be sought.

Movement	Two uses	Two effects
Effleurage	**To distribute the oil** **To relax the receiver** **of the massage**	**Improves blood and** **lymphatic circulation** **Soothes nerve endings**
Pétrissage	**To stimulate sluggish** **circulation** **To ease muscular** **tension**	**Erythema (redness)** **is produced** **Speeds up elimination** **of toxins**
Tapotement	**To invigorate the client** **To increase blood** **circulation**	**Erythema is produced** **Muscle fibres** **stimulated so muscle** **tone is improved**
Friction	**To invigorate the client** **To warm the area for** **deeper massage**	**Creates warmth in area** **worked** **Relieves tension in** **muscles**
Frictions	**To break down knots** **To relieve tension in** **muscles**	**Breaks down knots** **Releases muscular** **tension**
Vibration	**To stimulates sluggish** **lymphatic drainage** **To relieve tension**	**Relieves pain and** **fatigue** **Relieves tiredness** **and lethargy**

1. ◊ Relaxes muscles
   ◊ Increases blood circulation
   ◊ Increases lymphatic circulation
   ◊ Stimulates sebum secretion
   ◊ Stimulates sweat glands.
2. An increased circulation to the scalp will speed up cell division and ensure that more oxygen and nutrients are delivered to the skin and hair, which will improve their condition.
3. Will loosen scalp muscles and so relieve tension within them
   Oils condition and moisturise dry hair and scalp.
4. ◊ Ensure client's clothing is protected
   ◊ Be careful not to pour oil into the client's eyes
   ◊ Ensure that the client is not allergic to oil.
5. ◊ **Sesame oil –** thick, yellow liquid that is extracted from sesame seeds.
   ◊ **Mustard oil –** strong-smelling, thick, yellow liquid extracted from seeds of the mustard plant.
   ◊ **Olive oil –** thick, yellow/green oil extracted from the flesh of the olive.
   ◊ **Coconut oil –** light, cream-coloured oil extracted from the dried flesh of the coconut.
6. Effleurage, pétrissage, tapotement and vibrations massage movements.

Indian head massage element	Type of massage movement
Iron down	**Effleurage**
Finger kneading around scapulae	**Pétrissage**
Heel-of-hand knead around scapulae	**Pétrissage**
Hacking to upper back	**Tapotement**
Shoulder pick-up and squeeze	**Pétrissage**
Thumb push to shoulders	**Pétrissage**
Circular thumb knead to shoulders	**Pétrissage**
Pick-up and squeeze to upper arms	**Pétrissage**
Heel-of-hand circles to upper arms	**Pétrissage**
Knuckling to upper arms	**Pétrissage**
Fingers-and-thumb slide	**Effleurage**
Finger-and-heel-of-hand grasp to neck	**Pétrissage**
Eye circles with middle finger	**Effleurage**
Finger-and-thumb squeeze along jawbone	**Pétrissage**
Circular finger kneading to jaw bone	**Pétrissage**

1. ◆ Headache
   ◆ Dizziness
   ◆ Nausea
   ◆ Disrupted sleep pattern
   ◆ Increased mucous in nose or mouth.
2. Rest and relax after treatment
   Drink plenty of water or herbal teas to help detoxify the body
   Avoid drinks containing caffeine
   Do not drink alcohol or smoke for about 24 hours
   Eat light meals.
3. Regularly brush hair to help distribute sebum
   Protect hair from the sun and wear a cap when swimming
   Do not overuse hairdryers, heated rollers or curling tongs
   Avoid chemical processes, such as bleaching or perming
   Use conditioning treatments containing keratin
   Eat a well-balanced diet and drink plenty of water.
4. To ensure that the client gets the maximum benefit from the
   Indian head massage treatment.

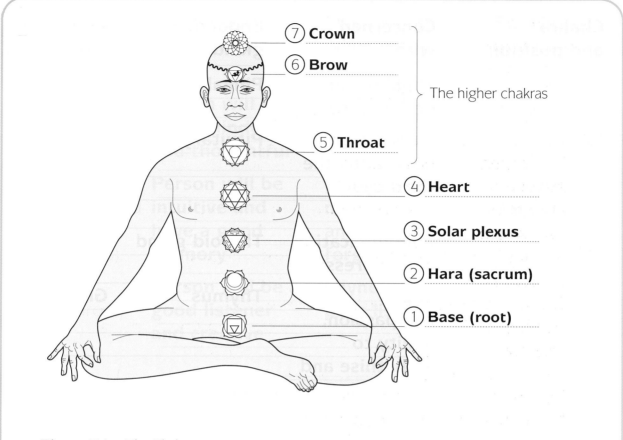

Figure 7.1 *The Chakras*